THE Lazy DIET

Lose Weight with Little Effort

By Norman P Lawson

Disclaimer

The information contained in this publication is intended to be educational and not for diagnosis, prescription, or treatment of any health disorder whatsoever. This publication was written with the understanding that neither the author nor publisher is engaged in rendering any medical or psychological advice. Readers should consult their physician prior to beginning a new exercise program, changing their diet, or making other lifestyle changes.

The publisher and author disclaim personal liability, directly or indirectly, for the information presented within this publication.

Although the author and publisher have prepared these manuscripts with utmost care and diligence and have made every effort to ensure the accuracy and completeness of the information contained within, we assume no responsibility for errors, inaccuracies, omissions, or inconsistencies.

Contents

Quick Start guide   113

Introduction

Its time to embrace your inner couch potato and start using your laziness to your advantage. The Lazy Diet is meant to be easy, especially for those of us who are lazy. This diet takes what some might consider as a weaknesses and turns it into something positive. If you take all of those imperfections that prevent most of us from succeeding at maintaining a healthy habits and you start using them to your advantage, you'll find that its not as hard as your thought to lose and ultimately maintain a healthy weight.

Being lazy is not a bad thing and if you want to be successful with your new diet you need to start looking at your current habits differently. The focus instead needs to be which activities could you benefit from being lazy? For example being too lazy to make that trip to the fridge or that drive to the store to buy junk food is not a bad thing.

Old habits die hard. Changing your habits is a process that involves several stages. Sometimes it takes a while before changes become new habits. And, you may face roadblocks along the way, but adopting new, healthier habits may protect you from serious health problems like obesity and diabetes. New habits, like healthy eating and regular physical activity, may also help you manage your weight and have more energy. After a while, if you stick with these changes, they may become part of your daily routine.

Fundamentals of Weight Loss

Your weight is a balancing act, and calories are part of that equation. Weight loss comes down to burning more calories than you take in. You can do that by reducing extra calories from food and beverages, and increasing calories burned through physical activity.

While that seems simple, it can be challenging to implement a practical, effective and sustainable weight-loss plan.

But you don't have to do it alone. Talk to your doctor, family and friends for support. Ask yourself if now is a good time and if you're ready to make some necessary changes. Also, plan smart: Anticipate how you'll handle situations that challenge your resolve and the inevitable minor setbacks.

If you have serious health problems because of your weight, your doctor may suggest weight-loss surgery or medications for you. In this case, your doctor will discuss the potential benefits and the possible risks with you.

But don't forget the bottom line: The key to successful weight loss is a commitment to making changes in your diet and exercise habits.

It's natural for anyone trying to lose weight to want to lose it very quickly. But evidence shows that people who lose weight gradually and steadily (about 1 to 2 pounds per week) are more successful at keeping weight off. Healthy weight loss isn't just about a "diet" or "program". It's about an ongoing lifestyle that includes long-term changes in daily eating and exercise habits.

Once you've achieved a healthy weight, by relying on healthful eating and physical activity most days of the week (about 60—90 minutes, moderate intensity), you are more likely to be successful at keeping the weight off over the long term.

Losing weight is not easy, and it takes commitment. But if you're ready to get started, we've got a step-by-step guide to help get you on the road to weight loss and better health.

Even modest weight loss can mean big benefits

The good news is that no matter what your weight loss goal is, even a modest weight loss, such as 5 to 10 percent of your total body weight, is likely to produce health benefits, such as improvements in blood pressure, blood cholesterol, and blood sugars.1

For example, if you weigh 200 pounds, a 5 percent weight loss equals 10 pounds, bringing your weight down to 190 pounds. While this weight may still be in the "overweight" or "obese" range, this modest weight loss can decrease your risk factors for chronic diseases related to obesity.

So even if the overall goal seems large, see it as a journey rather than just a final destination. You'll learn new eating and physical activity habits that will help you live a healthier lifestyle. These habits may help you maintain your weight loss over time.

In addition to improving your health, maintaining a weight loss is likely to improve your life in other ways. For example, a study of participants in the National Weight Control Registry* found that those who had maintained a significant weight loss reported improvements in not only their physical health, but also their energy levels, physical mobility, general mood, and self-confidence.

The Balance of Calories and Exercise

Our bodies need energy to keep us alive and our organs functioning normally. When we eat and drink, we put energy into our bodies. Our bodies use up that energy through everyday movement, which includes everything from breathing to running.

To maintain a stable weight, the energy we put into our bodies must be the same as the energy we use by normal bodily functions and physical activity. An important part of a healthy diet is balancing the energy you put into your bodies with the energy you use. For example, the more physical activity we do the more energy we use. If you consume too much energy on one day, don't worry; just try to take in less energy on the following days.

The amount of calories people use by doing a certain physical activity varies, depending on a range of factors, including size and age.

The more vigorously you do an activity, the more calories you will use. For example, fast walking will burn more calories than walking at a moderate pace.

If you're gaining weight, it could mean you've been regularly eating and drinking more calories than you've been using. To lose weight, you need to use more energy than you consume, and continue this over a period of time. The best approach is to combine diet changes with increased physical activity. Find out more about how much physical activity you should be doing.

Choosing the Right Foods

A healthy lifestyle involves many choices. Among them, choosing a balanced diet or healthy eating plan. So how do you choose a healthy eating plan? Let's begin by defining what a healthy eating plan is.

According to the Dietary Guidelines for Americans 2015-2020, a healthy eating plan:

- Emphasizes fruits, vegetables, whole grains, and fat-free or low-fat milk and milk products

- Includes lean meats, poultry, fish, beans, eggs, and nuts

- Is low in saturated fats, trans fats, cholesterol, salt (sodium), and added sugars

- Stays within your daily calorie needs

A healthy eating plan that helps you manage your weight includes a variety of foods you may not have considered. If "healthy eating" makes you think about the foods you can't have, try refocusing on all the new foods you can eat.

Fresh, Frozen, or Canned Fruits — don't think just apples or bananas. All fresh, frozen, or canned fruits are great choices. Be sure to try some "exotic" fruits, too. How about a mango? Or a juicy pineapple or kiwi fruit! When your favorite fresh fruits aren't in season, try a frozen, canned, or dried variety of a fresh fruit you enjoy. One caution about canned fruits is that they may contain added sugars or syrups. Be sure and choose canned varieties of fruit packed in water or in their own juice.

Fresh, Frozen, or Canned Vegetables — try something new. You may find that you love grilled vegetables or steamed vegetables with an herb you haven't tried like rosemary. You can sauté (pan fry) vegetables in a non-stick pan with a small amount of cooking spray. Or try frozen or canned vegetables for a quick side dish — just microwave and serve. When trying canned vegetables, look for vegetables without added salt, butter, or cream sauces. Commit to going to the produce department and trying a new vegetable each week.

Calcium-rich foods — you may automatically think of a glass of low-fat or fat-free milk when someone says "eat more dairy products." But what about low-fat and fat-free yogurts without added sugars? These come in a wide variety of flavors and can be a great dessert substitute for those with a sweet tooth.

A new twist on an old favorite — if your favorite recipe calls for frying fish or breaded chicken, try healthier variations using baking or grilling. Maybe even try a recipe that uses dry beans in place of higher-fat meats. Ask around or search the internet and magazines for recipes with fewer calories, you might be surprised to find you have a new favorite dish!

Healthy eating is all about balance. You can enjoy your favorite foods even if they are high in calories, fat or added sugars. The key is eating them only once in a while, and balancing them out with healthier foods and more physical activity.

Some general tips for comfort foods:

- Eat them less often. If you normally eat these foods every day, cut back to once a week or once a month. You'll be cutting your calories because you're not having the food as often.

- Eat smaller amounts. If your favorite higher-calorie food is a chocolate bar, have a smaller size or only half a bar.

- Try a lower-calorie version. Use lower-calorie ingredients or prepare food differently. For example, if your macaroni and cheese recipe uses whole milk, butter, and full-fat cheese, try remaking it with non-fat milk, less butter, light cream cheese, fresh spinach and tomatoes. Just remember to not increase your portion size. For more ideas on how to cut back on calories, see Eat More Weigh Less.

- The point is, you can figure out how to include almost any food in your healthy eating plan in a way that still helps you lose weight or maintain a healthy weight.

Exercise vs cutting back on calories

In addition to a healthy eating plan, an active lifestyle will help you maintain your weight. By choosing to add more physical activity to your day, you'll increase the amount of calories your body burns. This makes it more likely you'll maintain your weight.

Although physical activity is an integral part of weight management, it's also a vital part of health in general. Regular physical activity can reduce your risk for many chronic diseases and it can help keep your body healthy and strong.

Regular physical activity is important for good health, and it's especially important if you're trying to lose weight or to maintain a healthy weight.

When losing weight, more physical activity increases the number of calories your body uses for energy or "burns off." The burning of calories through physical activity, combined with reducing the number of calories you eat, creates a "calorie deficit" that results in weight loss.

Most weight loss occurs because of decreased caloric intake. However, evidence shows the only way to maintain weight loss is to be engaged in regular physical activity. Most importantly, physical activity reduces risks of cardiovascular disease and diabetes beyond that produced by weight reduction alone.

When it comes to weight management, people vary greatly in how much physical activity they need. Here are some guidelines to follow:

To maintain your weight: Work your way up to 150 minutes of moderate-intensity aerobic activity, 75 minutes of vigorous-intensity aerobic activity, or an equivalent mix of the two each week. Strong scientific evidence shows that physical activity can help you maintain your weight over time. However, the exact amount of physical activity needed to do this is not clear since it varies greatly from person to person. It's possible that you may need to do more than the equivalent of 150 minutes of moderate-intensity activity a week to maintain your weight.

To lose weight and keep it off: You will need a high amount of physical activity unless you also adjust your diet and reduce the amount of calories you're eating and drinking. Getting to and staying at a healthy weight requires both regular physical activity and a healthy eating plan.

Moderate: While performing the physical activity, if your breathing and heart rate is noticeably faster but you can still carry on a conversation — it's probably moderately intense. Examples include:

- Walking briskly (a 15-minute mile).

- Light yard work (raking/bagging leaves or using a lawn mower).

- Light snow shoveling.

- Actively playing with children.

- Biking at a casual pace.

Vigorous: Your heart rate is increased substantially and you are breathing too hard and fast to have a conversation, it's probably vigorously intense. Examples include:

- Jogging/running.

- Swimming laps.

- Roller blading / in-line skating at a brisk pace.

- Cross-country skiing.

- Most competitive sports (football, basketball, or soccer).

- Jumping rope.

The 4 pillars of weight loss

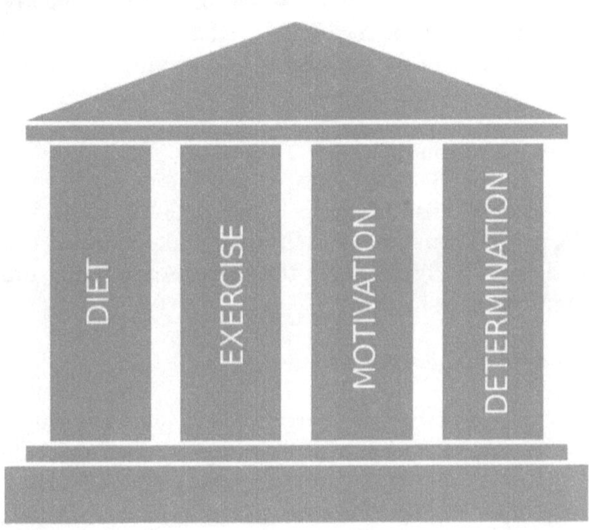

Diet

There is more than one way to eat healthfully and everyone has their own eating style. Make healthier choices that reflect your preferences, culture, traditions, and budget. Choose fruits, vegetables, grains, dairy, and protein foods to get the most nutrition and meet your personal calorie needs. Aim for a variety of foods and beverages from each food group and limit saturated fat, sodium, and added sugars.

The saturated fat, sodium, and added sugars found in foods and beverages are important for you to think about as you build your healthy eating style. Saturated fat and sodium are sometimes found naturally in foods and beverages. Sugars, sodium, and ingredients high in saturated fat can also be added during processing or preparing foods and beverages.

Create an eating style that can improve your health now and in the future by making small changes over time. Consider changes that reflect your personal preferences, culture and traditions. Think of each change as a "win" as you build positive habits and find solutions that reflect your healthy eating style. Each change should be an improvement that can help you build your healthy eating style. Use the tips below to find little victories that work for you.

Try to choose a variety of foods and beverages from each food group to build healthy eating styles. Include choices from all the food groups to meet your calorie and nutrient needs when planning or preparing meals and snacks.

Many weight loss diets promise to help you lose weight quickly. Often these diets only focus on short-term results, so you eventually end up putting the weight back on. Here are five reasons why following the latest novelty diet may not be a good way to lose weight.

1. Some diets can make you ill

Many diets, especially crash diets, are geared to dramatically reducing the number of calories you consume. Crash diets make you feel very unwell and unable to function properly, because they are nutritionally unbalanced and can lead to long-term poor health

2. Excluding foods is dangerous

Some diets recommend cutting out certain foods, such as meat, fish, wheat or dairy products. Cutting out certain food groups altogether could prevent you getting the important nutrients and vitamins your body needs to function properly. You can lose weight without cutting out foods from your diet.

3. Low-carb diets can be high in fat

Some diets, such as the Atkins diet, are very low in carbohydrates (for example, pasta, bread and rice), which are an important source of energy. While you may lose weight on these types of diets, they're often high in protein and fat, which can make you ill. Low-carbohydrate diets can also cause side effects such as bad breath, headaches and constipation.

Many low-carbohydrate diets allow you to eat foods high in saturated fat, such as butter, cheese and meat. Too much saturated fat can raise your cholesterol and increase your risk of heart disease and stroke.

4. Detox diets don't work

Detox diets are based on the idea that toxins build up in the body and can be removed by eating, or not eating, certain things. However, there's no evidence that toxins build up in our bodies. If they did, we would feel very ill. Detox diets may lead to weight loss because they involve restricting calories, cutting out certain foods altogether, such as wheat or dairy, and eating a very limited range of foods.

5. Cabbage soup, blood group, the 5:2 diet and other fad diets are often far-fetched

Some fad diets are based on eating a single food or meal, such as cabbage soup or raw foods. Others make far-fetched claims, such as encouraging people to cut out certain foods from their diet based on their blood type.

Intermittent fasting, which includes the increasingly popular 5:2 diet, is a pattern of eating where you eat normally five days a week and fast on the other two days. Fans of the 5:2 diet say it can help you live longer and protect you against disease. Often there is little or no evidence to back up these claims, and it can be difficult to keep to in the long term.

Exercise

Regular physical activity will not only help you lose weight, but could also reduce your risk of developing a serious illness.

The amount of physical activity that is recommended depends on your age. Adults aged 19 to 64 who are new to activity should aim to build up to 150 minutes of moderate-intensity aerobic activity a week.

Our bodies need energy to keep us alive and our organs functioning normally. When we eat and drink, we put energy into our bodies. Our bodies use up that energy through everyday movement, which includes everything from breathing to running.

To maintain a stable weight, the energy we put into our bodies must be the same as the energy we use by normal bodily functions and physical activity. An important part of a healthy diet is balancing the energy you put into your bodies with the energy you use. For example, the more physical activity we do the more energy we use. If you consume too much energy on one day, don't worry; just try to take in less energy on the following days.

Motivation

Losing weight takes more than desire. It takes commitment and a well-thought-out plan. Here's a step-by-step guide to getting started.

Step 1: Make a commitment.

Making the decision to lose weight, change your lifestyle, and become healthier is a big step to take. Start simply by making a commitment to yourself. Many people find it helpful to sign a written contract committing to the process. This contract may include things like the amount of weight you want to lose, the date you'd like to lose the weight by, the dietary changes you'll make to establish healthy eating habits, and a plan for getting regular physical activity.

Writing down the reasons why you want to lose weight can also help. It might be because you have a family history of heart disease, or because you want to see your kids get married, or simply because you want to feel better in your clothes. Post these reasons where they serve as a daily reminder of why you want to make this change.

Step 2: Take stock of where you are.

Consider talking to your health care provider. He or she can evaluate your height, weight, and explore other weight-related risk factors you may have. Ask for a follow-up appointment to monitor changes in your weight or any related health conditions.

Keep a "food diary" for a few days, in which you write down everything you eat. By doing this, you become more aware of what you are eating and when you are eating. This awareness can help you avoid mindless eating.

Next, examine your current lifestyle. Identify things that might pose challenges to your weight loss efforts. For example, does your work or travel schedule make it difficult to get enough physical activity? Do you find yourself eating sugary foods because that's what you buy for your kids? Do your coworkers frequently bring high-calorie items, such as dough nuts, to the workplace to share with everyone? Think through things you can do to help overcome these challenges.

Finally, think about aspects of your lifestyle that can help you lose weight. For example, is there an area near your workplace where you and some coworkers can take a walk at lunchtime? Is there a place in your community, such as a YMCA, with exercise facilities for you and child care for your kids?

Step 3: Set realistic goals.

Set some short-term goals and reward your efforts along the way. If your long-term goal is to lose 40 pounds and to control your high blood pressure, some short-term eating and physical activity goals might be to start eating breakfast, taking a 15 minute walk in the evenings, or having a salad or vegetable with supper.

Focus on two or three goals at a time. Great, effective goals are:

- Specific

- Realistic

- Forgiving (less than perfect)

For example, "Exercise More" is not a specific goal. But if you say, "I will walk 15 minutes, 3 days a week for the first week," you are setting a specific and realistic goal for the first week.

Remember, small changes every day can lead to big results in the long run. Also remember that realistic goals are achievable goals. By achieving your short-term goals day-by-day, you'll feel good about your progress and be motivated to continue. Setting unrealistic goals, such as losing 20 pounds in 2 weeks, can leave you feeling defeated and frustrated.

Being realistic also means expecting occasional setbacks. Setbacks happen when you get away from your plan for whatever reason – maybe the holidays, longer work hours, or another life change. When setbacks happen, get back on track as quickly as possible. Also take some time to think about what you would do differently if a similar situation happens, to prevent setbacks.

Keep in mind everyone is different – what works for someone else might not be right for you. Just because your neighbor lost weight by taking up running, doesn't mean running is the best option for you. Try a variety of activities – walking, swimming, tennis, or group exercise classes to see what you enjoy most and can fit into your life. These activities will be easier to stick with over the long term.

Step 4: Identify resources for information and support.

Find family members or friends who will support your weight loss efforts. Making lifestyle changes can feel easier when you have others you can talk to and rely on for support. You might have coworkers or neighbors with similar goals, and together you can share healthful recipes and plan group exercise. Joining a weight loss group or visiting a health care professional such as a registered dietitian or nutritionist, can help.

Step 5: Continually "check in" with yourself to monitor your progress.

Revisit the goals you set for yourself (in Step 3) and evaluate your progress regularly. If you set a goal to walk each morning but are having trouble fitting it in before work, see if you can shift your work hours or if you can get your walk in at lunchtime or after work. Evaluate which parts of your plan are working well and which ones need tweaking. Then rewrite your goals and plan accordingly. If you are consistently achieving a particular goal, add a new goal to help you continue on your pathway to success.

Reward yourself for your successes! Recognize when you're meeting your goals and be proud of your progress. Use non-food rewards, such as a bouquet of freshly picked flowers, a sports outing with friends, or a relaxing bath. Rewards help keep you motivated on the path to better health.

Determination

Set the Right Goals

Setting the right goals is an important first step. Most people trying to lose weight focus on just that one goal: weight loss. However, the most productive areas to focus on are the dietary and physical activity changes that will lead to long-term weight change. Successful weight managers are those who select two or three goals at a time that are manageable.

Useful goals should be (1) specific; (2) attainable (doable); and (3) forgiving (less than perfect). "Exercise more" is a great goal, but it's not specific. "Walk 5 miles every day" is specific and measurable, but is it doable if you're just starting out? "Walk 30 minutes every day" is more attainable, but what happens if you're held up at work one day and there's a thunderstorm during your walking time another day? "Walk 30 minutes, 5 days each week" is specific, doable, and forgiving. In short, a great goal!

Nothing Succeeds Like Success

Shaping is a behavioral technique in which you select a series of short-term goals that get closer and closer to the ultimate goal (e.g., an initial reduction of fat intake from 40 percent of calories to 35 percent of calories, and later to 30 percent). It is based on the concept that "nothing succeeds like success." Shaping uses two important behavioral principles: (1) consecutive goals that move you ahead in small steps are the best way to reach a distant point; and (2) consecutive rewards keep the overall effort invigorated.

Reward Success (But Not With Food)

An effective reward is something that is desirable, timely, and dependent on meeting your goal. The rewards you choose may be material (e.g., a movie or music CD, or a payment toward buying a more costly item) or an act of self-kindness (e.g., an afternoon off from work or just an hour of quiet time away from family). Frequent small rewards, earned for meeting smaller goals, are more effective than bigger rewards that require a long, difficult effort.

Balance Your Food Checkbook

"Self-monitoring" refers to observing and recording some aspect of your behavior, such as calorie intake, servings of fruits and vegetables, amount of physical activity, etc., or an outcome of these behaviors, such as weight. Self-monitoring of a behavior can be used at times when you're not sure how you're doing, and at times when you want the behavior to improve. Self-monitoring of a behavior usually moves you closer to the desired direction and can produce "real-time" records for review by you and your health care provider. For example, keeping a record of your physical activity can let you and your provider know quickly how you're doing. When the record shows that your activity is increasing, you'll be encouraged to keep it up. Some patients find that specific self-monitoring forms make it easier, while others prefer to use their own recording system.

While you may or may not wish to weigh yourself frequently while losing weight, regular monitoring of your weight will be essential to help you maintain your lower weight. When keeping a record of your weight, a graph may be more informative than a list of your weights. When weighing yourself and keeping a weight graph or table, however, remember that one day's diet and exercise patterns won't have a measurable effect on your weight the next day. Today's weight is not a true measure of how well you followed your program yesterday, because your body's water weight will change from day to day, and water changes are often the result of things that have nothing to do with your weight-management efforts.

Avoid a Chain Reaction

Stimulus (cue) control involves learning what social or environmental cues seem to encourage undesired eating, and then changing those cues. For example, you may learn from reflection or from self-monitoring records that you're more likely to overeat while watching television, or whenever treats are on display by the office coffee pot, or when around a certain friend. You might then try to change the situation, such as by separating the association of eating from the cue (don't eat while watching television), avoiding or eliminating the cue (leave the coffee room immediately after pouring coffee), or changing the circumstances surrounding the cue (plan to meet your friend in a nonfood setting). In general, visible and reachable food items are often cues for unplanned eating.

Get the Fullness Message

Changing the way you go about eating can make it easier to eat less without feeling deprived. It takes 15 or more minutes for your brain to get the message that you've been fed. Eating slowly will help you feel satisfied. Eating lots of vegetables and fruits can make you feel fuller. Another trick is to use smaller plates so that moderate portions do not appear too small. Changing your eating schedule, or setting one, can be helpful, especially if you tend to skip, or delay, meals and overeat later.

Watch Your Diet

Follow a healthy and realistic eating pattern. You have embarked on a healthier lifestyle, now the challenge is maintaining the positive eating habits you've developed along the way. In studies of people who have lost weight and kept it off for at least a year, most continued to eat a diet lower in calories as compared to their pre-weight loss diet.

Keep your eating patterns consistent. Follow a healthy eating pattern regardless of changes in your routine. Plan ahead for weekends, vacations, and special occasions. By making a plan, it is more likely you'll have healthy foods on hand for when your routine changes.

Eat breakfast every day. Eating breakfast is a common trait among people who have lost weight and kept it off. Eating a healthful breakfast may help you avoid getting "over-hungry" and then overeating later in the day.

Get daily physical activity. People who have lost weight and kept it off typically engage in 60—90 minutes of moderate intensity physical activity most days of the week while not exceeding calorie needs. This doesn't necessarily mean 60—90 minutes at one time. It might mean 20—30 minutes of physical activity three times a day. For example, a brisk walk in the morning, at lunch time, and in the evening. Some people may need to talk to their health care provider before participating in this level of physical activity.

Stay on Course:

Monitor your diet and activity. Keeping a food and physical activity journal can help you track your progress and spot trends. For example, you might notice that your weight creeps up during periods when you have a lot of business travel or when you have to work overtime. Recognizing this tendency can be a signal to try different behaviors, such as packing your own healthful food for the plane and making time to use your hotel's exercise facility when you are traveling. Or if working overtime, maybe you can use your breaks for quick walks around the building.

Monitor your weight. Check your weight regularly. When managing your weight loss, it's a good idea to keep track of your weight so you can plan accordingly and adjust your diet and exercise plan as necessary. If you have gained a few pounds, get back on track quickly.

Get support from family, friends, and others. People who have successfully lost weight and kept it off often rely on support from others to help them stay on course and get over any "bumps." Sometimes having a friend or partner who is also losing weight or maintaining a weight loss can help you stay motivated.

The Perfect "LAZY" Diet

We put on weight when the amount of calories we eat exceeds the amount of calories we burn through normal everyday activities and exercise. *Most adults just need to eat less and get more active!*

The only way to lose weight healthily and keep it off is to make permanent changes to the way you eat and exercise. A few small alterations, such as eating less and choosing drinks that are lower in fat, sugar and alcohol, can help you lose weight. There are also plenty of ways to make physical activity part of your life.

Calculating your Basal Metabolic Rate (BMR)

First to calculate your BMR using the formulas below. This will tell you how many calories you need to consume to maintain your current weight with little to no activity or exercise.

- Women: BMR = 655 + (4.35 x weight in pounds) + (4.7 x height in inches) - (4.7 x age in years)

- Men: BMR = 66 + (6.23 x weight in pounds) + (12.7 x height in inches) - (6.8 x age in years)

Next use the formulas below based on different levels of activity. This will also give you an idea how different levels of activities change the amount of calories you can consume. Multiply your BMR by the appropriate activity factor, as follows:

- Sedentary (little or no exercise): BMR x 1.2

- Lightly active (light exercise/sports 1-3 days/week): BMR x 1.375

- Moderately active (moderate exercise/sports 3-5 days/week): BMR x 1.55

- Very active (hard exercise/sports 6-7 days a week): BMR x 1.725

Extra active (very hard exercise/sports & physical job or 2x training): BMR x 1.9

The BMR calculates the maximum number of calories you consume, in order to lose weight you will need to consume less than that amount. It is suggested that you consume no less than 75% of the calculated BMR to maintain a healthy weight-loss plan. You don't want to lose weight too quickly because the goal of any new diet should be to change your eating habits and maintain those habits for a long time. If you consume too little calories you are just creating another bad habit and one that will be unhealthy to maintain.

Finding Healthy Substitutes

Eating fewer calories doesn't necessarily mean eating less food. To be able to cut calories without eating less and feeling hungry, you need to replace some higher calorie foods with foods that are lower in calories and   fill you up. In general, these foods contain a lot of water and are high in fiber.

Most people try to reduce their calorie intake by focusing on food, but another way to cut calories may be to change what you drink. You may find that you're consuming quite a few calories just in the beverages you have each day. Find out how you can make better drink choices to reduce your calorie intake.

You may find that your portion sizes are leading you to eat more calories than you realize. Research shows that people unintentionally consume more calories when faced with larger portions. This can mean excessive calorie intake, especially when eating high-calorie foods.

Learn about fruits and vegetables and their role in your weight management plan. Tips to cut calories by substituting fruits and vegetables are included with meal-by-meal examples. You will also find snack ideas that are 100 calories or less. With these helpful tips, you will soon be on your way to adding more fruits and vegetables into your healthy eating plan.

Breakfast	Substitution	Calories Reduced by
Top your cereal with low fat or fat-free milk instead of 2% or whole milk.	1 cup of fat-free milk instead of 1 cup of whole milk	63
Use a non-stick pan and cooking spray (rather than butter) to scramble or fry eggs	1 spray of cooking spray instead of 1 pat of butter	34
Choose reduced-calorie margarine spread for toast rather than butter or stick margarine.	2 pats of reduced calorie margarine instead of 2 pats of butter	36
Lunch	**Substitution**	**Calories**

		Reduced by
Add more vegetables such as cucumbers, lettuce, tomato, and onions to a sandwich instead of extra meat or cheese.	2 slices of tomatoes, ¼ cup of sliced cucumbers, and 2 slices of onions instead of an extra slice (3/4 ounce) of cheese and 2 slices (1 ounce) of ham	154
Accompany a sandwich with salad or fruit instead of chips or French fries.	½ cup diced raw pineapple instead of 1 ounce bag of potato chips	118
Choose vegetable-based broth soups rather than cream- or meat-based soups.	1 cup of vegetable soup instead of 1 cup cream of chicken soup	45
When eating a salad, dip your fork into dressing instead of pouring lots of dressing on the salad.	½ TBSP of regular ranch salad dressing instead of 2 TBSP of regular ranch dressing	109
When eating out, substitute a broth-based soup or a green lettuce salad for French fries or chips as a side dish	A side salad with a packet of low-fat vinaigrette dressing instead of a medium order of French fries	270

Dinner	Substitution	Calories Reduced by
Have steamed or grilled vegetables rather than those sautéed in butter or oil. Try lemon juice and herbs to flavor the vegetables. You can also sauté with non-stick cooking spray.	½ cup steamed broccoli instead of ½ cup broccoli sautéed in 1/2 TBSP of vegetable oil.	62
Modify recipes to reduce the amount of fat and calories. For example, when making lasagna, use part-skim	1 cup of part-skim ricotta cheese instead of 1 cup whole milk ricotta cheese	89

ricotta cheese instead of whole-milk ricotta cheese. Substitute shredded vegetables, such as carrots, zucchini, and spinach for some of the ground meat in lasagna.

When eating out, have a cocktail or dessert instead of both during the same eating occasion.	Choosing one or the other saves you calories. A 12-ounce beer has about 153 calories. A slice of apple pie (1/6 of a 8″ pie) has 277 calories.	153
When having pizza, choose vegetables as toppings and just a light sprinkling of cheese instead of fatty meats.	One slice of a cheese pizza instead of one slice of a meat and cheese pizza	60

Snacks	Substitution	Calories Reduced by
Choose air-popped popcorn instead of oil-popped popcorn and dry-roasted instead of oil-roasted nuts.	3 cups of air-popped popcorn instead of 3 cups of oil-popped popcorn	73
Avoid the vending machine by packing your own healthful snacks to bring to work. For example, consider vegetable sticks, fresh fruit, low fat or nonfat yogurt without added sugars, or a small handful of dry-roasted nuts.	An eight-ounce container of no sugar added nonfat yogurt instead of a package of 6 peanut butter crackers	82
Choose sparkling water instead of sweetened drinks or alcoholic beverages.	A bottle of carbonated water instead of a 12-ounce can of soda with sugar	136

Instead of cookies or other sweet snacks, have some fruit for a snack.

One large orange instead of 3 chocolate sandwich cookies — 54

Selecting the right foods

A healthy eating plan gives your body the nutrients it needs every day while staying within your daily calorie goal for weight loss. A healthy eating plan also will lower your risk for heart disease and other health conditions.

To reduce the time you spend in the kitchen, you can improve your organization by using a shopping list and keeping a well-stocked pantry. Shop for quick, low-fat food items, and fill your kitchen cupboards with a supply of low-calorie basics.

Read labels as you shop. Pay attention to the serving size and the servings per container. All labels list total calories in a serving size of the product. Compare the total calories in the product you choose with others like it; choose the one that is lowest in calories. Below is a sample Nutrition Facts label that identifies important information.

- Emphasizes vegetables, fruits, whole grains, and fat-free or low-fat dairy products

- Includes lean meats, poultry, fish, beans, eggs, and nuts

- Limits saturated and trans fats, sodium, and added sugars

- Controls portion sizes

Prepare a list of the groceries you need ahead of time and stick to the list when you go to the store. This will keep you focused and can help prevent any spur of the moment, high calorie purchases.

Learning From the Label

First, look at the serving size and number of servings.

Then, look at calories, total fat, saturated fat, cholesterol, and sodium per serving.

The "% Daily Value" shows you how much of the recommended amounts the food provides in one serving, if you eat 2,000 calories a day. For example, one serving of this food gives you 5 percent of your total fat recommendation.

At the bottom of the label, you can see the recommended daily amount for each nutrient for two calorie levels (2,000 and 2,500 calorie diets)

Nutrition Facts

Serving Size 2/3 cup (55g)
Servings Per Container About 8

Amount Per Serving

Calories 230	Calories from Fat 72

	% Daily Value*
Total Fat 8g	**12%**
Saturated Fat 1g	**5%**
Trans Fat 0g	
Cholesterol 0mg	**0%**
Sodium 160mg	**7%**
Total Carbohydrate 37g	**12%**
Dietary Fiber 4g	**16%**
Sugars 12g	
Protein 3g	
Vitamin A	10%
Vitamin C	8%
Calcium	20%
Iron	45%

* Percent Daily Values are based on a 2,000 calorie diet. Your daily value may be higher or lower depending on your calorie needs.

	Calories:	2,000	2,500
Total Fat	Less than	65g	80g
Sat Fat	Less than	20g	25g
Cholesterol	Less than	300mg	300mg
Sodium	Less than	2,400mg	2,400mg
Total Carbohydrate		300g	375g
Dietary Fiber		25g	30g

Nutrition Facts

8 servings per container

Serving size	**2/3 cup (55g)**

Amount per serving

Calories	**230**

	% Daily Value*
Total Fat 8g	**10%**
Saturated Fat 1g	**5%**
Trans Fat 0g	
Cholesterol 0mg	**0%**
Sodium 160mg	**7%**
Total Carbohydrate 37g	**13%**
Dietary Fiber 4g	**14%**
Total Sugars 12g	
Includes 10g Added Sugars	**20%**
Protein 3g	
Vitamin D 2mcg	10%
Calcium 260mg	20%
Iron 8mg	45%
Potassium 235mg	6%

* The % Daily Value (DV) tells you how much a nutrient in a serving of food contributes to a daily diet. 2,000 calories a day is used for general nutrition advice.

Slipping from your diet

It is not uncommon for people who have lost weight to start slipping back into old behaviors and seeing their weight slowly creep up. That said, just because it is not uncommon does not mean it is inevitable!

A lapse might be overeating during dinner for a day or two, or skipping your physical activity for a week while you are on vacation. Lapses are a natural part of weight management. At some point, everyone has lapses – small slips, moments, or brief periods of time when they return to an old habit.

A lapse left unchecked, however, can grow into a relapse. A relapse usually results from a series of several small lapses that snowball into a full-blown relapse. The most effective way to prevent a relapse is to identify the lapses early and deal with them before they turn into a relapse.

A lapse (or a single occasion of uncontrolled eating or not being physically active) is not likely – by itself – to cause you to slip back into old habits and regain weight. However, when people eat something they know they shouldn't or stop being active, they often have self-defeating thoughts.

Step 1: The first step in dealing with lapses is to recognize that 99.9% of all people trying to lose weight and be active experience lapses. Lapses can and should be useful learning experiences.

Step 2: The second step is to resist the tendency to think negative thoughts. You are not a failure if you lapse – you are normal!

Step 3: Next, ask yourself what happened. Use the chance to learn from the lapse. Was it a special occasion? If so, is it likely to happen again soon? Did you eat because of social pressure? Did you skip physical activity because you were too busy with other things, or because of work and family pressures? Review the situation and think about it neutrally. Then plan a strategy for dealing more effectively with similar situations in the future.

Step 4: The fourth step is to regain control of your eating or physical activity at the very next opportunity. Do not tell yourself, "Well, I blew it for the day," and wait until the next day to get back on track. Getting back on track without delay is important in preventing lapses from becoming relapses.

Step 5: Talk to someone supportive. Call your Lifestyle Coach, another participant, or another friend or loved one and discuss your new strategy for handling lapses. Step 6: Finally, remember you are making life-long changes. Weight loss is a journey with lots of small decisions and choices every day that add up over time. Focus on all the positive changes you have made and realize that you can get back on track.

In addition, situations may not be high-risk across the board. A situation that makes you want to eat high-calorie foods may not affect your physical activity routine, and vice versa. Also consider what situations seem to decrease your self-monitoring behavior, which is an easy way to start slipping on eating and activity. Finally, remember that both positive and negative situations can be risky for lapses. Think about times in the past several weeks when you might have slipped or had a lapse. What was going on? What circumstances led to your lapse? There are some situations that are commonly identified as high-risk by individuals trying to manage their weight. Review the categories on the following worksheet: emotional, routine, social, and other. Circle those that apply to you, and write in your own high-risk situations.

Your plan should involve taking action to change the situation, your thoughts and behaviors, or both. Make sure your plan is specific and detailed, so that you will be able to follow it when you are in the middle of a high-risk situation.

Having a lapse is a natural part of weight management. Even when you have an excellent plan to handle your slips and high-risk situations, you cannot always prevent or avoid lapses. This does not mean you have failed or that you will regain your weight. Keep these things in mind while planning your comeback:

- Reflect on your progress. Remember your purpose.

- Remember that a short period of overeating or skipped activity will not erase all of your progress.

- Be kind to yourself. Stay calm and listen to your positive self-talk (while sending away negative thoughts). How you think about your lapse is the most important part of the process. If you use it as a learning opportunity, you will succeed. If you give up and stop trying to make changes, then you are at risk for a relapse.

Think about what will be the most effective comeback plan for you to recover from a lapse and prevent a full relapse. Write down these steps and keep your written plan in a place where you can easily find it when you need it.

1. What two steps can I take immediately after a lapse to get back on track.

2. What negative thinking might get in the way of putting my comeback plan into action?

3. What positive thoughts will I use to keep myself going with my comeback plan?

4. How will I reward myself when I get back on track?

Foods to watch out for

The saturated fat, sodium, and added sugars found in foods and beverages are important for you to think about as you build your healthy eating style. Saturated fat and sodium are sometimes found naturally in foods and beverages. Sugars, sodium, and ingredients high in saturated fat can also be added during processing or preparing foods and beverages.

To reduce your risk for heart disease, cut back on saturated fat and trans fat by replacing some foods high in saturated fat with unsaturated fat or oils.

SATURATED FAT

Imagine a building made of solid bricks. This building of bricks is similar to the tightly packed bonds that make "saturated" fat. The bonds are often solid at room temperature like butter or the fat inside or around meat. Saturated fats are most often found in animal products such as beef, pork, and chicken. Leaner animal products, such as chicken breast or pork loin, often have less saturated fat. Foods that contain more saturated fat are usually solid at room temperature and are sometimes called "solid" fat.

UNSATURATED FAT

Now, imagine the links in a chain that bend, move, and flow. The chain links are similar to the loose bonds that make "unsaturated" fat fluid or liquid at room temperature like the oil on top of a salad dressing or in a can of tuna. Unsaturated fat typically comes from plant sources such as olives, nuts, or seeds – but unsaturated fat is also present in fish. Unsaturated fat are usually called oils. Unlike saturated fat, these oils contain mostly monounsaturated and polyunsaturated fat.

A few food products such as coconut oil, palm oils, or whole milk remain as liquids at room temperature but are high in saturated fat.

TRANS FAT

Trans fat can be made from vegetable oils through a process called hydrogenation**. Trans fat is naturally found in small amounts in some animal products such as meat, whole milk, and milk products. Check the food label to find out if trans fat is in your food choices. Trans fat can often be found in many cakes, cookies, crackers, icings, margarines, and microwave popcorn.

LIMIT SATURATED AND TRANS FAT

Eating more unsaturated fat than saturated and trans fats can reduce your risk of heart disease and improve "good" (HDL) cholesterol levels. Replace foods high in saturated and trans fat such as butter, whole milk, and baked goods with foods higher in unsaturated fat found in plants and fish, such as vegetable oils, avocado, and tuna fish.

SOME COMMON FOODS CONTAINING SATURATED FAT

beef fat (tallow, suet)   butter   chicken fat

Cut back on foods containing saturated fat including:

- desserts and baked goods, such as cakes, cookies, donuts, pastries, and croissants

- many cheeses and foods containing cheese, such as pizza

- sausages, hot dogs, bacon, and ribs

- ice cream and other dairy desserts

- fried potatoes (French fries) – if fried in a saturated fat or hydrogenated oil

- regular ground beef and cuts of meat with visible fat

- fried chicken and other chicken dishes with the skin

- whole milk and full-fat dairy foods

OILS AS PART OF A HEALTHY EATING STYLE

Oils provide essential fatty acids and vitamin E. They are found in different plants such as soybeans, olives, corn, sunflowers, and peanuts. Choosing unsaturated oils instead of saturated fat can help you maintain a healthy eating style. A few plant oils, including coconut and palm oil, are higher in saturated fat and should be eaten less often.

- Choose foods higher in unsaturated fat and lower in saturated fat as part of your healthy eating style.

- Use oil-based dressings and spreads on foods instead of butter, stick margarine, or cream cheese.

- Drink fat-free (skim) or low-fat (1%) milk instead of reduced-fat (2%) or whole milk.

- Buy lean cuts of meat instead of fatty meats or choose these foods less often.

- Add low-fat cheese to homemade pizza, pasta, and mixed dishes.

- In recipes, use low-fat plain yogurt instead of cream or sour cream.

SODIUM

Most of us get more sodium than we need. While adding salt to your food is a source of sodium, it may not be the main reason that your sodium intake is high. Packaged and prepared foods such as ready-to-eat products or restaurant meals are common sources of sodium.

Sodium is added to packaged foods during processing such as in curing meat, baking, thickening, enhancing flavor, as a preservative, or to keep foods moist.

ADDED SUGARS

Added sugars are sweeteners and syrups that are added when foods or beverages are processed or prepared. Many foods and beverages contain calories from added sugars. Added sugars can make a food or beverage tastier, but they can also add a lot of calories and few or no nutrients. Most adults eat or drink about 18 teaspoons of added sugar each day.

Choosing an eating style with less added sugars and more nutrient-dense foods can help you manage your calories.

To build a healthy eating style and stay within your calorie needs, choose foods and beverages with less added sugars. Added sugars are sugars and syrups that are added to foods or beverages when they are processed or prepared. This does not include natural sugars found in milk and fruits.

Most of us eat and drink too many added sugars from the following foods:

beverages, such as regular soft drinks, energy or sports drinks, fruit drinks, sweetened coffee and tea

- candy

- cakes

- cookies and brownies

- pies and cobblers

- sweet rolls, pastries, and donuts

- ice cream and dairy desserts

- sugars, jams, syrups, and sweet toppings

Creating good habits

When it comes to eating, we have strong habits. Some are good ("I always eat breakfast"), and some are not so good ("I always clean my plate"). Although many of our eating habits were established during childhood, it doesn't mean it's too late to change them.

Making sudden, radical changes to eating habits such as eating nothing but cabbage soup, can lead to short term weight loss. However, such radical changes are neither healthy nor a good idea, and won't be successful in the long run. Permanently improving your eating habits requires a thoughtful approach in which you Reflect, Replace, and Reinforce.

REFLECT on all of your specific eating habits, both bad and good; and, your common triggers for unhealthy eating.

REPLACE your unhealthy eating habits with healthier ones.

REINFORCE your new, healthier eating habits.

Create a list of your eating habits. Keeping a food diary for a few days, in which you write down everything you eat and the time of day you ate it, will help you uncover your habits. For example, you might discover that you always seek a sweet snack to get you through the mid-afternoon energy slump. It's good to note how you were feeling when you decided to eat, especially if you were eating when not hungry. Were you tired? Stressed out?

Highlight the habits on your list that may be leading you to overeat. Common eating habits that can lead to weight gain are:

- Eating too fast

- Always cleaning your plate

- Eating when not hungry

- Eating while standing up (may lead to eating mindlessly or too quickly)

- Always eating dessert

- Skipping meals (or maybe just breakfast)

Look at the unhealthy eating habits you've highlighted. Be sure you've identified all the triggers that cause you to engage in those habits. Identify a few you'd like to work on improving first. Don't forget to pat yourself on the back for the things you're doing right. Maybe you almost always eat fruit for dessert, or you drink low-fat or fat-free milk. These are good habits! Recognizing your successes will help encourage you to make more changes.

Create a list of "cues" by reviewing your food diary to become more aware of when and where you're "triggered" to eat for reasons other than hunger. Note how you are typically feeling at those times. Often an environmental "cue", or a particular emotional state, is what encourages eating for non-hunger reasons.

Common triggers for eating when not hungry are:

- Opening up the cabinet and seeing your favorite snack food.

- Sitting at home watching television.

- Before or after a stressful meeting or situation at work.

- Coming home after work and having no idea what's for dinner.

- Having someone offer you a dish they made "just for you!"

- Walking past a candy dish on the counter.

- Sitting in the break room beside the vending machine.

- Seeing a plate of doughnuts at the morning staff meeting.

- Swinging through your favorite drive-through every morning.

- Feeling bored or tired and thinking food might offer a pick-me-up.

Circle the "cues" on your list that you face on a daily or weekly basis. Going home for the Thanksgiving holiday may be a trigger for you to overeat, and eventually, you want to have a plan for as many eating cues as you can. But for now, focus on the ones you face more often.

Ask yourself these questions for each "cue" you've circled:

Is there anything I can do to avoid the cue or situation? This option works best for cues that don't involve others. For example, could you choose a different route to work to avoid stopping at a fast food restaurant on the way? Is there another place in the break room where you can sit so you're not next to the vending machine?

For things I can't avoid, can I do something differently that would be healthier? Obviously, you can't avoid all situations that trigger your unhealthy eating habits, like staff meetings at work. In these situations, evaluate your options. Could you suggest or bring healthier snacks or beverages? Could you offer to take notes to distract your attention? Could you sit farther away from the food so it won't be as easy to grab something? Could you plan ahead and eat a healthy snack before the meeting?

Replace unhealthy habits with new, healthy ones. For example, in reflecting upon your eating habits, you may realize that you eat too fast when you eat alone. So, make a commitment to share a lunch each week with a colleague, or have a neighbor over for dinner one night a week. Other strategies might include putting your fork down between bites or minimizing other distractions (i.e. watching the news during dinner) that might keep you from paying attention to how quickly — and how much — you're eating.

Here are more ideas to help you replace unhealthy habits:

Eat more slowly. If you eat too quickly, you may "clean your plate" instead of paying attention to whether your hunger is satisfied.

Eat only when you're truly hungry instead of when you are tired, anxious, or feeling an emotion besides hunger. If you find yourself eating when you are experiencing an emotion besides hunger, such as boredom or anxiety, try to find a non-eating activity to do instead. You may find a quick walk or phone call with a friend helps you feel better.

Plan meals ahead of time to ensure that you eat a healthy well-balanced meal.

Reinforce your new, healthy habits and be patient with yourself. Habits take time to develop. It doesn't happen overnight. When you do find yourself engaging in an unhealthy habit, stop as quickly as possible and ask yourself: Why do I do this? When did I start doing this? What changes do I need to make? Be careful not to berate yourself or think that one mistake "blows" a whole day's worth of healthy habits. You can do it! It just takes one day at a time!

Exercise

When and how often to exercise

It is up to you, but it is better to spread your activity throughout the week and to be active at least 3 days a week.

It's your choice. Pick an activity that's easy to fit into your life. Do at least 10 minutes of physical activity at a time. Choose aerobic activities that work for you. These make your heart beat faster and can make your heart, lungs, and blood vessels stronger and more fit. Also do strengthening activities which make your muscles do more work than usual.

Do a little more each time. Once you feel comfortable, do it more often. Then, you can trade activities at a moderate level for vigorous ones that take more effort. You can do moderate and vigorous activities in the same week.

Physical activity can make you feel stronger and more alive. It is a fun way to be with your family or friends. It also helps you improve your health.

Perfect exercises for beginners

Light Activities	Moderate Activities	Vigorous Activities
Casual Walking	Ballroom dancing	Aerobic dance
Walking up stairs	Biking on level ground	Biking
Golf	Canoeing	Rock Climbing
Child Care	General gardening	Hiking uphill
Household Cleaning	Tennis	Jumping rope
Mild Stretching	Using hand cyclers	Running
Shopping	Walking briskly	Basketball
Mowing Grass	Water aerobics	Swimming

Perfect exercises for those with little time

Sometimes rules about healthy behaviors can feel ingrained. However, there are some creative ways people can find time for health-benefiting movement in shorter time periods. Add these into your next patient conversation about physical activity.

Build in activity breaks. Try to avoid inactivity by regularly building in activity time. Set a timer on your watch, or use an app on your phone to remind you to get up and move every hour.

Be creative. People can get active wherever they go. Counsel patients and clients to consider creative ways to squeeze in activity – even on a business trip or to their child's soccer game. For example, a Tabata circuit (8 rounds of 20 seconds of activity and 10 second of rest) could be done with exercises like lunges, push ups, jumping jacks, sit ups, and more. Several circuits can be done in a hotel room on a business trip. On the sidelines, parents could select an exercise and complete it every time a goal is scored or the ball changes teams. They could also jog around the field – either steady state, or in intervals with walking and jogging or running, during half time. Another idea: people can try a new workout app; some highlight sessions as short as seven minutes, which can easily be used on the go.

Find options that work. Fitness facilities in the area often offer day passes or a la carte classes, and in areas near a lot of businesses, some classes are as short as 30 minutes. For many people, paying ahead of time for a class can add additional motivation to follow through and attend.

Incorporate exercise into everyday play. Ten minutes spent playing tag as a family is a great way to get in some extra movement.

Be active on the go. When you're out and about walking, parking farther away, or getting off the bus/train a stop early can add a few more minutes of activity to the day.

Replacing daily activities

One of the best ways to add more exercise to your schedule is to replace daily activities with something that is more physically demanding. These can be easy activities like taking the stairs instead of an elevator or using a push mower instead of a riding lawn mower. You'll find that they don't have to be big changes to have a significant impact on your health and how you feel.

Calories Used per Hour in Common Physical Activities

Moderate Physical Activity	Approximate Calories/30 Minutes for a 154 lb Person1	Approximate Calories/Hr for a 154 lb Person1
Hiking	185	370
Light gardening/yard work	165	330
Dancing	165	330
Golf (walking and carrying clubs)	165	330
Bicycling (<10 mph)	145	290
Walking (3.5 mph)	140	280
Weight lifting (general light workout)	110	220
Stretching	90	180

Vigorous Physical Activity	Approximate Calories/30 Minutes for a 154 lb Person1	Approximate Calories/Hr for a 154 lb Person1
Running/jogging (5 mph)	295	590
Bicycling (>10 mph)	295	590
Swimming (slow freestyle laps)	255	510
Aerobics	240	480
Walking (4.5 mph)	230	460

Heavy yard work (chopping wood)	220	440
Weight lifting (vigorous effort)	220	440
Basketball (vigorous)	220	440

Working Out at Home

It's usually convenient, comfortable and safe to work out at home. It allows your children to see you being active, which sets a good example for them. You can combine exercise with other activities, such as watching TV. If you buy exercise equipment, it's a one-time expense and other family members can use it. It's easy to have short bouts of activity several times a day.

Try these tips:

- Do housework yourself instead of hiring someone else to do it.

- Work in the garden or mow the grass. Using a riding mower doesn't count! Rake leaves, prune, dig and pick up trash.

- Go out for a short walk before breakfast, after dinner or both! Start with 5-10 minutes and work up to 30 minutes.

- Walk or bike to the corner store instead of driving.

When walking, pick up the pace from leisurely to brisk. Choose a hilly route. When watching TV, sit up instead of lying on the sofa. Or stretch. Better yet, spend a few minutes pedaling on your stationary bicycle while watching TV. Throw away your video remote control. Instead of asking someone to bring you a drink, get up off the couch and get it yourself.

- Stand up while talking on the telephone.

- Walk the dog.

- Park farther away at the shopping mall and walk the extra distance. Wear your walking shoes and sneak in an extra lap or two around the mall.

- Stretch to reach items in high places and squat or bend to look at items at floor level.

- Keep exercise equipment repaired and use it!

Working Out at Work

Many of us have sedentary jobs, and work takes up a significant part of our day. What can you do to increase your physical activity during the work day? Why not...:

- Brainstorm project ideas with a coworker while taking a walk.

- Create an exercise accountability partnership.

- Walk during business calls when you don't need to reference important documents.

- Stand while talking on the telephone.

- Walk down the hall to speak with someone rather than using the telephone.

- Take the stairs instead of the elevator. Or get off a few floors early and take the stairs the rest of the way.

- Walk while waiting for the plane at the airport.

- Stay at hotels with fitness centers or swimming pools and use them while on business trips.

- Take along a jump rope or a resistance band in your suitcase when you travel. Jump and do calisthenics in your hotel room.

- Download some audio fitness coaching.

- Participate in or start a recreation league at your company.

- Form a sports team to raise money for charity events.

- Join a fitness center or YMCA near your job. Work out before or after work to avoid rush-hour traffic, or drop by for a noon workout.

- Schedule exercise time on your business calendar and treat it as any other important appointment.

- Get off the bus a few blocks early and walk the rest of the way to work or home.

- Walk around your building for a break during the work day or during lunch.

- Some have mastered the art of typing while on a treadmill by securing the laptop to the base. Be creative!

- Get a stand-up desk.

Play and Recreation

Play and recreation are important for good health. Look for opportunities such as these to be active and have fun at the same time:

- Plan family outings and vacations that include physical activity (hiking, backpacking, swimming, etc.)

- See the sights in new cities by walking, jogging or bicycling.

- Make a date with a friend to enjoy your favorite physical activities. Do them regularly.

- Play your favorite music while exercising; enjoy something that motivates you.

- Dance with someone or by yourself. Take dancing lessons. Hit the dance floor on fast numbers instead of slow ones.

- Join a recreational club that emphasizes physical activity.

- At the beach, sit and watch the waves instead of lying flat. Better yet, get up and walk, run or fly a kite.

- When golfing, walk instead of using a cart.

- Play singles tennis or racquetball instead of doubles.

- At a picnic, join in on badminton instead of croquet.

- At the lake, rent a rowboat instead of a canoe.

Helpful tips

To reduce the amount of fat you eat, you could trim the fat off meat, drink skimmed or semi-skimmed milk instead of full fat, choose a reduced- or low-fat spread, and replace cream with low-fat or Greek yogurt. Find out about some more healthy food swaps.

Eat wholegrain foods, such as wholemeal bread, brown rice and pasta. They're digested more slowly than the white varieties, so will help you feel full for longer.

Don't skip breakfast. A healthy breakfast will give you the energy you need to start the day, and there's some evidence that people who eat breakfast regularly are less likely to be overweight.

Aim to eat at least five portions of a variety of fruit and vegetables a day.]

If you feel like a snack, try having a drink first, such as a glass of water or cup of tea. Often we think we're hungry when really we're thirsty.

Swap drinks high in calories for lower calorie alternatives – that means drinks that are lower in fat, sugars and alcohol. Swap a sugary fizzy drink for sparkling water with a slice of lemon. Don't forget that alcohol is high in calories, so cutting down on alcohol can help you control your weight.

1. Don't skip breakfast

Skipping breakfast won't help you lose weight. You could miss out on essential nutrients and you may end up snacking more throughout the day because you feel hungry. Check out five healthy breakfasts.

2. Eat regular meals

Eating at regular times during the day helps burn calories at a faster rate. It also reduces the temptation to snack on foods high in fat and sugar.

3. Eat plenty of fruit and veg

Fruit and veg are low in calories and fat, and high in fiber – 3 essential ingredients for successful weight loss. They also contain plenty of vitamins and minerals.

4. Get more active

Being active is key to losing weight and keeping it off. As well as providing numerous health benefits, exercise can help burn off the excess calories you can't cut through diet alone. Find an activity you enjoy and are able to fit into your routine.

5. Drink plenty of water

People sometimes confuse thirst with hunger. You can end up consuming extra calories when a glass of water is really what you need.

6. Eat high-fiber foods

Foods containing lots of fiber can help keep you to feel full, which is perfect for losing weight. Fiber is only found in food from plants, such as fruit and veg, oats, wholegrain bread, brown rice and pasta, and beans, peas and lentils.

7. Read food labels

Knowing how to read food labels can help you choose healthier options. Use the calorie information to work out how a particular food fits into your daily calorie allowance on the weight loss plan. Find out more about reading food labels.

8. Use a smaller plate

Using smaller plates can help you eat smaller portions. By using smaller plates and bowls, you may be able to gradually get used to eating smaller portions without going hungry. It takes about 20 minutes for the stomach to tell the brain it's full, so eat slowly and stop eating before you feel full.

9. Don't ban foods

Don't ban any foods from your weight loss plan, especially the ones you like. Banning foods will only make you crave them more. There's no reason you can't enjoy the occasional treat as long as you stay within your daily calorie allowance.

10. Don't stock junk food

To avoid temptation, try to not stock junk food – such as chocolate, biscuits, crisps and sweet fizzy drinks – at home. Instead, opt for healthy snacks, such as fruit, unsalted rice cakes, oat cakes, unsalted or unsweetened popcorn, and fruit juice.

11. Cut down on alcohol

A standard glass of wine can contain as many calories as a piece of chocolate. Over time, drinking too much can easily contribute to weight gain. Find out more about the calories in alcohol.

12. Plan your meals

Try to plan your breakfast, lunch, dinner and snacks for the week, making
sure you stick to your calorie allowance. You may find it helpful to make a
weekly shopping list.

Norman P Lawson

38

Recipes

Apple Oatmeal Muffins

Calories: 125 per serving

Ingredients

- 1/2 cup milk, non-fat
- 1/3 cup applesauce
- 1/2 cup flour, all-purpose
- 1/2 cup quick-cooking oats (uncooked)
- 1/4 cup sugar
- 1/2 tablespoon baking powder
- 1/2 teaspoon ground cinnamon
- 1 apple (tart, cored & chopped)

Directions

1. Preheat oven to 400°F.

2. Place 6 cupcake holders in baking tin.

3. In a mixing bowl, add milk and applesauce. Stir until blended.

4. Stir in flour, oats, sugar, baking powder, and cinnamon. Mix until moistened (do not over mix).

5. Gently stir in the chopped apples.

6. Spoon into cupcake holders.

7. Bake for 15-20 minutes or until an inserted toothpick comes out clean.

8. Cool in pan 5 minutes before serving. Store unused portions in an airtight container

Apple Slice Pancakes

Calories: 174 per serving

Ingredients

- 1 apple (Granny Smith)
- 1 1/4 cups pancake mix (any type)
- 1/2 teaspoon cinnamon
- 1 large egg
- 2 teaspoons canola oil
- 1 cup milk, low-fat

Directions

1. Lightly coat a griddle or skillet with cooking spray and heat over medium heat.

2. Peel, core and thinly slice apple into rings.

3. In a large mixing bowl, combine ingredients for pancake batter. Stir until ingredients are evenly moist. (Small lumps are ok! Over-mixing makes pancakes tough.)

4. For each pancake, place apple ring on griddle and pour about 1/4 cup batter over apple ring, starting in the center and covering the apple.

5. Cook until bubbles appear. Turn and cook other side until lightly brown.

Notes

To test the griddle to see if it is hot, sprinkle it with a few drops of water. When the drops sizzle and dance, you are ready to cook! The easiest way to pour the batter onto the hot griddle is to use a 1/4 cup measuring cup for each pancake. If the first pancake is too brown, lower the heat.

Banana Oat Muffins

Calories: 160 per serving

Ingredients

- 2 cups oat circles cereal (crushed)
- nonstick cooking spray
- 1 1/4 cups flour
- 1/3 cup packed brown sugar (or 1/3 cup regular sugar)
- 1 teaspoon baking powder
- 3/4 teaspoon baking soda
- 2 medium ripe bananas (mashed)
- 2/3 cup 1% milk
- 3 tablespoons vegetable oil
- 1 egg

Directions

1. Preheat oven to 400 degrees F.
2. Spray 12 regular-sized muffin cups with nonstick cooking spray, or line cups with paper muffin cup liners.
3. Mix cereal, flour, brown sugar, baking powder, and baking soda in a large bowl.
4. Add bananas, milk, oil, and egg.
5. Stir just until moistened.
6. Divide batter among 12 muffin cups.
7. Bake 18 to 22 minutes until golden brown.

Notes

You may use 2 to 3 bananas for this recipe.

Banana Split Oatmeal

Calories: 267per serving

Ingredients

- 1/3 cup oatmeal (dry, quick-cooking)
- 1/8 teaspoon salt
- 3/4 cup water (very hot)
- 1/2 banana (sliced)
- 1/2 cup frozen yogurt (non-fat)

Directions

1. In a microwave safe cereal bowl, mix together the oatmeal and salt. Stir in water.
2. Microwave on high power for 1 minute. Stir. Microwave on high power for another minute. Stir again.
3. Microwave an additional 30-60 seconds on high power until the cereal reaches the desired thickness. Stir again.
4. Top with banana slices and frozen yogurt.

Notes

The banana split oatmeal can be a snack by itself.

Banana Waldorf

Calories: 312 per serving

Makes: 4 servings

Sweetened with bananas and apples, this recipe makes a healthy dessert, a satisfying afternoon snack, or even a tasty breakfast.

Ingredients

- 3 banana (peeled and sliced)
- 1 apple (cored and sliced, with peel)
- 4 cups yogurt (nonfat vanilla)
- 1/16 teaspoon cinnamon (pinch)
- 1/8 cup walnuts (ground)

Directions

1. 1. Mix all ingredients together in large mixing bowl.
2. 2. Place in individual serving dishes and chill until ready to serve, up to 1 hour.
3. 3. This dessert looks great when topped with a sprinkle of ground cinnamon.

Basic Quiche

You can vary this recipe by using whatever vegetables you have on hand (fresh, frozen, or canned)!

Calories: 133 per serving

Makes: 6 servings

Ingredients

- 1 pie crust (baked, 9-inch)
- 1 cup vegetables (chopped, broccoli, zucchini, or mushrooms)
- 1/2 cup cheese (shredded)
- 3 egg (beaten)
- 1 cup milk (non-fat)
- 1/2 teaspoon salt
- 1/2 teaspoon pepper
- 1/2 teaspoon garlic powder

Directions

1. Preheat the oven to 375 degrees.
2. Shred the cheese with a grater. Put it in a small bowl for now.
3. Chop the vegetables until you have 1 cup of chopped vegetables.
4. Cook the vegetables until they are cooked, but still crisp.
5. Put the cooked vegetables and shredded cheese into a pie shell.
6. Mix the eggs, milk, salt, pepper, and garlic powder in a bowl.
7. Pour the egg mix over the cheese and vegetables
8. Bake for 30-40 minutes, or until a knife inserted near the center comes out clean.
9. Let the quiche cool for 5 minutes before serving

Breakfast Burrito

The protein and fiber in this bean, vegetable, and yogurt breakfast burrito make great additions to your morning meal.

Calories 146 per serving

Serving Size 1 Burrito

Ingredients

- 1 1/3 cups black beans (cooked, mashed with 1 teaspoon canola oil, or use canned vegetarian refried beans)
- 4 tortillas, corn
- 2 tablespoons red onion (chopped)
- 1/2 cup tomatoes (chopped)
- 1/2 cup salsa, low-sodium
- 4 tablespoons yogurt, non-fat plain
- 2 tablespoons cilantro (chopped)

Directions

1. Mix beans with onion and tomatoes.
2. Microwave tortillas between the two sheets of slightly damp white paper towels on high for 15 seconds.
3. Divide bean mixture between the tortillas.
4. Fold each tortilla to enclose filling.
5. Place on microwave-safe dish and spoon salsa over each burrito.
6. Microwave on high for 15 seconds.
7. Serve topped with yogurt and cilantro.

Breakfast Parfait

This colorful parfait features four types of fruit: fresh, frozen, canned, and dried.

Calories: 209 per serving

Makes 4 Servings

Ingredients

- 2 cups pineapple, canned and chopped
- 1 cup berries, frozen (thawed)
- 1 cup yogurt, low-fat vanilla
- 1 banana (peeled and sliced)
- 1/3 cup raisins

Directions

1. In glasses or bowls, layer pineapple, berries, yogurt, banana, and raisins.

Broccoli-Cheddar Frittata

Calories: 160 per serving

Makes 6 servings

Ingredients

- 1 package (10-oz) frozen chopped broccoli
- 1/4 cup water
- 8 eggs
- 1/4 cup nonfat or low-fat milk
- 2 teaspoons prepared mustard
- 1 teaspoon seasoned salt
- 1/8 teaspoon pepper
- 3/4 cup shredded reduced-fat cheddar cheese (3 oz)
- 1 tablespoon Chopped green onion
- 1 small carrot, diced
- nonstick cooking spray

Directions

1. Combine broccoli, carrot, if desired, and water in 10-inch nonstick skillet. Cook over medium heat until tender, stirring occasionally to break up broccoli, about 10 minutes; drain well.

2. Beat eggs, milk, mustard, salt and pepper in large bowl until blended. Add broccoli mixture, cheese and green onion; mix well.

3. Coat same skillet with cooking spray; heat over medium heat until eggs are almost set, 8 to 10 minutes.

4. Remove from heat. Cover and let stand until eggs are completely set and no visible liquid egg remains, 8 to 10 minutes. Cut into wedges.

Notes

Broil option: After removing from heat, frittata can be broiled, 6 inches from heat until eggs are completely set and no visible liquid egg remains, 2 to 3 minutes.

Green Onion Omelet

In the spring, in areas where they grow, wild onions can be used in place of green onions. Yellow or white onions work as well.

Calories: 184 per serving

Makes 4 servings

Ingredients

- 1 can low-sodium sliced potatoes (drained, about 15 ounces)
- 1 tablespoon vegetable oil
- 1 egg (whole)
- 3 egg whites
- 3 tablespoons 1% low-fat milk
- 1/4 teaspoon salt
- 1/2 cup ham (diced)
- 1/2 can low-sodium tomatoes (drained, about 8 ounces)
- 1 tablespoon green onion or wild onion (chopped)

Directions

1. Open and drain can of sliced potatoes. Cut sliced potatoes into strips.
2. In a large skillet over medium heat, lightly brown potatoes in the vegetable oil for 5 to 10 minutes.
3. In a mixing bowl, add egg, egg whites, milk, and salt. Mix well
4. Stir in ham, tomatoes, and green (or wild) onions.
5. Pour egg mixture over potatoes in the skillet.
6. Cover skillet and continue to cook eggs over medium heat until firm, not runny (about 8 minutes).
7. Cut the omelet into four pieces and serve.

Herbed Spinach Quiche Portabella Caps

Calories: 190 per serving

Makes 4 servings

Ingredients

- 4 portabella mushrooms (3-inch diameter)
- cooking spray
- 3 large eggs
- 6 egg whites from 6 eggs
- 1/2 cup whole-wheat grated bread crumbs
- 1/4 cup nonfat milk
- 1 teaspoon low-sodium garlic & herb blend
- 1 cup cooked and drained, chopped, frozen spinach
- 1/4 cup reduced-fat Parmesan cheese, divided

Directions

1. Place oven rack in center of oven; preheat oven to 375 °F.
2. Remove portabella stems; wipe clean with damp paper towel.
3. Spray baking sheet with cooking spray, and place mushroom caps on baking sheet.
4. In a mixing bowl, whisk together all remaining ingredients, except 1 tbsp Parmesan cheese.
5. Coat 10-inch non-stick pan with cooking spray and heat over medium flame.
6. Cook and scramble egg mixture until it just starts to thicken. Remove from heat.
7. Using a large spoon, scoop partially cooked, hot egg mixture into portabella caps.
8. Sprinkle tops with remaining Parmesan cheese. Bake about 20 minutes.

Microwave Denver Scramble Slider

This quick egg scramble sandwich is made fast in the microwave for a great on-the-go breakfast, lunch or snack.

Calories: 240 per serving

Makes 1 serving

Ingredients

- 2 tablespoons chopped red or green bell peppers
- 1 tablespoon chopped onion
- 1 egg
- 1 thin slice deli ham (chopped)
- 1 tablespoon water
- 1 slider-size bun or whole wheat English muffin (split and toasted)

Directions

1. 1. Place peppers and onions in 8-oz. ramekin or custard cup, or in a small bowl. Microwave on high 30 seconds; stir. Add egg, ham and water, beat until egg is blended.

2. 2. Microwave on high 30 seconds; stir. Microwave until egg is almost set, 30 to 45 seconds longer. Season with salt and pepper, if desired.

3. 3. Serve in bun.

Notes

Don't overcook. Scrambled eggs will continue to cook and firm up after removed from microwave.

Quesadilla con Huevos

Calories: 252 per serving

Makes 4 Servings

Makes 6 servings

Tortillas, eggs, cheese, and salsa can be enjoyed at any meal. Enjoy this main dish with a salad and a piece of fruit for a well balanced lunch.

Ingredients

- 1/2 cup cheddar or cojack cheese (grated)

- 2 egg (scrambled)

- 4 flour tortillas (6 - 8 inch)

- salsa (4 Tablespoons, optional)

Directions

1. Put 2 Tablespoons cheese and 1/4 of the scrambled eggs on each tortilla.

2. Heat 2 quesadillas at a time in microwave on high for 30 to 45 seconds or until cheese melts.

3. Top with salsa and fold tortilla in half to serve.

Notes

Kids can make these as plain as they like or can add ingredients such as peppers, tomatoes, mushrooms or onions. Quesadillas make a great breakfast or lunch that's easy and quick. Instead of using a microwave, you can heat the tortillas on a skillet or griddle until the cheese melts.

Spanish Omelet

Calories: 289 per serving

Makes 5 Servings

Ingredients

- 5 potatoes (small, peeled and sliced)
- 1 tablespoon olive oil (or vegetable cooking spray)
- 1/2 onion (medium, minced)
- 1 zucchini (medium, sliced)
- 1 1/2 cups green/red peppers (sliced thin)
- 5 mushrooms (medium, sliced)
- 3 eggs (whole, beaten)
- 5 egg whites (beaten)
- Pepper and garlic salt with herbs (to taste)
- 3 ounces part skim mozzarella cheese (shredded)
- 1 tablespoon Parmesan cheese

Directions

1. Preheat oven to 375°F.

2. Cook potatoes in boiling water until tender.

3. In a nonstick pan, add oil or vegetable spray and warm at medium heat.

4. Add the onion and sauté until brown. Add vegetables and sauté until tender but not brown.

5. In a medium mixing bowl, slightly beat the eggs and egg whites, pepper, garlic salt, and mozzarella cheese. Stir egg cheese mixture into the cooked vegetables.

6. Oil or spray a 10-inch pie pan or oven-proof skillet. Transfer potatoes and eggs mixture to pan. Spread with parmesan cheese and bake omelet until firm and brown on top, about 20-30 minutes.

Fiesta Wrap

Calories: 175 per serving

Makes 6 servings

Ingredients

- 1/4 cup Quinoa, dry
- 2 1/4 cups Canned low-sodium black beans, drained, rinsed
- 1/4 cup Fresh red bell pepper, seeded, diced
- 1/4 cup Fresh red onions, peeled, diced
- 1/2 cup Fresh carrots, peeled, diced
- 1/4 cup Reduced-fat white cheddar cheese, shredded (1 oz)
- 1 teaspoon chili powder
- 1 1/4 teaspoons ground cumin
- 1 1/4 teaspoons Fresh lime juice
- 6 Whole-wheat tortillas, 6"
- 1 tablespoon vegetable oil

Directions

1. Preheat oven to 325 °F.

2. Rinse quinoa in a fine mesh strainer until water runs clear, not cloudy. Combine quinoa and ¾ cup water in a small pot. Cover and bring to a boil. Turn heat down to low and simmer until water is completely absorbed, about 10-15 minutes. When done, quinoa will be soft and a white ring will pop out of the kernel.

3. Place black beans in a large mixing bowl. Lightly mash beans by squeezing them using gloved hands (at least 50 percent of the beans should appear whole). Be careful not to over-mash beans.

4. To make filling, add to the mashed beans the quinoa, red peppers, red onions, carrots, cheese, chili powder, cumin, and lime juice.

5. For each wrap, place ½ cup of filling on the bottom half of tortilla and roll in the form of a burrito. The wrap may also be folded in half like a taco.

6. Brush filled wraps lightly with vegetable oil and place on a baking sheet. Bake for 10 minutes at 325 °F. Wraps will be lightly brown.

Peanut, Peach, N Pineapple Wrap

Calories: 430 per serving

Makes 4 Servings

Ingredients

- 1 can sliced peaches (15 oz, drained)
- 1 can pineapple tidbits in juice (drained)
- 1/2 cup red or green bell pepper (chopped)
- 1 teaspoon cinnamon
- 4 whole wheat tortillas (10-inch)
- 1/2 cup chunky peanut butter
- 3 cups lettuce (shredded)

Directions

1. In a medium bowl, combine peaches, pineapple, bell pepper and cinnamon.
2. Warm the tortillas.
3. Spread 2 tablespoons of peanut butter on one side of each tortilla, leaving room on the edges.
4. Spoon equal portions of the peach mixture over peanut butter, then top with lettuce.
5. Fold the side and bottom edges of each tortilla toward the middle over the filling, then roll so the tortilla covers the filling.

Notes

Mix the drained juices with your breakfast juice if you like.

To make them more pliable before wrapping, warm tortillas. 10 to 15 seconds on high heat in the microwave, 3 to 5 minutes at 350ºF in aluminum foil in the oven, and 15 seconds per side over medium-high on the stove top.

Shake It Off with a Turkey Roll

Calories: 501 per serving

Makes 1 serving

Ingredients

- Fresh blueberries
- Fresh strawberries, sliced
- Fresh spinach, torn into bite-sized pieces
- Fresh romaine lettuce, torn into bite-sized pieces
- Carrot slivers
- 1 tablespoon ranch dressing
- 1 soft tortilla
- 1/4 teaspoon mayonnaise
- 2 slices turkey breast
- 1 slice Colby Jack cheese

Directions

1. Place the blueberries and strawberries in a small container together.

2. Place the spinach, romaine, and carrots in a small container together. Place the lid on the container and shake.

3. Place the ranch dressing in a small container (I like mine separate so my salad isn't soggy by lunchtime).

4. Place the tortilla on the cutting board. Spread mayonnaise on the tortilla, add the turkey, veggies, and cheese, roll the tortilla up, and cut it into 1-inch sections.

Tuna Slider with Green Chiles

Calories: 285 per serving

Makes 3 servings

Ingredients

- 5 ounces canned tuna, packed in water, drained and flaked

- 1 can chopped green chilies (1-4.25 oz. can)

- 1/4 cup diced celery

- 1/4 cup diced red onion

- 1/4 cup reduced fat mayonnaise

- 2 tablespoons chopped fresh cilantro or parsley

- 6 slider rolls, split

- Lettuce leaves

Directions

1. In large bowl combine tuna, green chilies, celery, red onion, mayonnaise and chopped cilantro; toss to mix well.

2. Top bottom half of each roll with lettuce leaves; top with some tuna mixture and top half of roll.

Apple Cranberry Salad Toss

Enjoy the best of fall flavors with this sweet and tart green salad. Light yet crisp, it's a perfect dish for the autumnal change of weather.

Calories: 174 per serving

Makes 8 servings

Ingredients

- 1 head of lettuce (about 10 cups)
- 2 apples (medium, sliced)
- 1/2 cup walnuts (chopped)
- 1 cup dried cranberries
- 1/2 cup green onion (sliced)
- 3/4 cup vinaigrette dressing

Directions

1. Toss lettuce, apples, walnuts, cranberries, and onions in a large bowl.

2. Add dressing; toss to coat. Serve immediately.

Broccoli Salad

Chopped broccoli, raisins, onion and crumbled bacon make this colorful salad a tasty side dish.

Calories: 174 per serving

Makes 8 servings

Ingredients

- 6 cups broccoli (chopped)
- 1 cup raisins
- 1 red onion (medium, peeled and diced)
- 2 tablespoons sugar
- bacon slices (8 slices, cooked and crumbled, optional)
- 2 tablespoons lemon juice
- 3/4 cup mayonnaise, low-fat

Directions

1. Combine all ingredients in a medium bowl.
2. Mix well.
3. Chill for 1 to 2 hours.
4. Serve.

Chicken and Cranberry Salad

A simple and delicious salad topped with almonds and dried cranberries for bursts of flavor.

Calories: 338 per serving

Makes 4 serving

Ingredients

- 12 ounces chicken, cooked and diced (1 1/2 cups)
- 1/2 cup vinaigrette dressing
- 1 cup dried cranberries (or cherries)
- 1/8 cup almonds (sliced)
- 1 head of lettuce (chopped)

Directions

1. Toss chicken, cranberries, and almonds with dressing.
2. Serve on a mound of chopped lettuce.

Chicken Pasta Salad

Colorful veggies, black beans, and pasta make this salad healthy, flavorful, and filling. Make it several hours ahead and let it chill in the refrigerator for a quick summer dinner.

Calories: 235 per serving

Makes 7 servings

Ingredients

- 2 cups cooked small pasta
- 1 1/2 cups canned chicken (drained)
- 1 cup diced bell pepper
- 1/2 cup sliced green onion
- 1 cup shredded yellow squash
- 1/2 cup canned corn kernels (drained)
- 1/2 cup frozen peas
- 1 can black beans, low sodium (15 oz, rinsed and drained)
- 1/2 cup fat-free Italian dressing

Directions

1. Cook pasta according to package directions, drain; rinse.
2. Combine first eight ingredients (pasta through black beans) in a large bowl.
3. Toss gently with salad dressing.
4. Chill for several hours to blend flavors.

Citrus Salad

This recipe to can help make half your plate fruits and vegetables. Grapefruit sections are a great addition to fruit or green salads.

Calories: 48 per serving

Makes 8 servings

Ingredients

- 1 grapefruit (peeled)
- 1 orange (peeled)
- 10 cups fresh greens (lettuce)
- 1 red onion (small, sliced thin)
- 2 tablespoons cider vinegar
- 1 tablespoon lime juice
- 1 tablespoon vegetable oil
- 1 tablespoon water
- 1/4 teaspoon black pepper
- 1/4 teaspoon cumin

Directions

1. Cut fruit into bite size pieces.
2. Toss with lettuce and onion. Mix remaining ingredients for dressing. Drizzle over salad and toss just before serving.

Cobb Salad with Pears

Sweet and savory, this Cobb Salad is sure to delight with the addition of canned pears, carrots, and Parmesan cheese.

Calories: 64 per serving

Makes 6 servings

Ingredients

For the Salad:

- 2 canned pear halves

- 6 cups Mesclun mix baby greens

- 1/2 tablespoon Parmesan cheese

- 1 1/3 cups carrots, grated

- 3 tablespoons walnuts

For the Dressing:

- 1/4 cup pear juice
- 1/4 teaspoon cider vinegar
- 1/4 teaspoon honey
- 1/4 teaspoon dijon mustard
- 1 dash salt and black pepper
- 1/4 teaspoon extra virgin olive oil

Directions

1. For the dressing, mix pear juice, vinegar, honey, mustard, and salt and pepper and olive oil in a blender.

2. Put mixed greens in large mixing bowl, drizzle dressing over greens and mix together.

3. Add remaining chopped pear,walnuts, and grated carrots and toss lightly.

4. Portion out 1 cup of salad and top with 1/2 tablespoon grated Parmesan cheese.

Cranberry Salad

Sweet strawberry gelatin and tart cranberry sauce make a yummy dish. Make ahead and keep in the refrigerator until ready to eat.

Calories: 267 per serving

Makes 10 servings

Ingredients

- 3 packages strawberry gelatin (3 oz. packages, can also use raspberry)
- 4 cups water
- 1 can cranberry sauce
- 1/4 cup sugar
- 2 tablespoons orange peel rind (grated)
- 2 tablespoons lemon juice
- 1 cup crushed pineapple (drained)
- 2 cups diced celery
- 3/4 cup walnuts

Directions

1. Make gelatin and refrigerate until partially set.
2. Beat cranberry sauce.
3. Grate orange peel into sugar and add to cranberry sauce with rest of ingredients.
4. Fold mixture into partially set gelatin. Refrigerate until set. Serve.

Notes

Suggested to serve with a mixture of instant lemon pudding mix and low-fat whipped topping.

Cucumber Blueberry Salad

A quick, simple and refreshing salad featuring fresh blueberries and crisp cucumber chunks with feta cheese, arugula and a lime vinaigrette.

Calories: 212 per serving

Makes 4 servings

Ingredients

Vinaigrette

- 1 1/2 tablespoons extra virgin olive oil
- 2 tablespoons white balsamic (or other) vinegar
- 1 tablespoon lime juice, freshly squeezed or bottled
- 1 teaspoon sugar
- 1/4 teaspoon salt
- 1/8 teaspoon pepper

Salad

- 1 cup fresh blueberries
- 1 medium greenhouse-grown cucumber, cut into small chunks
- 4 cups fresh arugula
- 1/4 medium red onion, thinly sliced
- 1/4 cup crumbled reduced-fat Feta cheese
- 2 tablespoons coarsely chopped walnuts (toasted optional)
- 4 slices whole grain bread

Directions

1. In a small bowl whisk together vinaigrette ingredients.
2. In a large bowl mix together all salad ingredients, except bread.
3. When ready to serve, add vinaigrette to salad and toss.
4. Toast bread, then cut into four pieces.

Easy Greek Salad

While feta cheese is the star of any Greek salad, this recipe contains all of the must-have ingredients for a classic salad that is sure to please.

Calories: 79 per serving

Makes 6 servings

Ingredients

- 6 romaine lettuces leaves (torn into 1 1/2 inch pieces)
- 1 cucumber (medium, peeled and sliced)
- 1 tomato (medium, chopped)
- 1/2 cup red onion (sliced)
- 1/3 cup feta cheese (crumbled)
- 2 tablespoons olive oil (extra-virgin)
- 2 tablespoons lemon juice
- 1 teaspoon oregano (dried)
- 1/2 teaspoon salt

Directions

1. Combine lettuce, cucumber, tomato, onion and cheese in large serving bowl. Whisk together oil, lemon juice, oregano and salt in small bowl.

2. Pour over lettuce mixture; toss until coated. Serve immediately.

Easy Summer Salad

Fresh red onion is used in this recipe. This Easy Summer Salad is great as a side dish for many meals.

Calories: 80 per serving

Makes 6 servings

Ingredients

- 1 cucumber (peeled and cut into small cubes)
- 1 red onion (peeled and cut into small cubes)
- 2 tomatoes (cut into small cubes)
- 1 clove garlic
- 4 tablespoons lemon juice
- 1 tablespoon vegetable oil
- 1/4 teaspoon salt
- black pepper (to taste)

Directions

1. Add cucumbers, onions, tomatoes, and garlic in a large bowl.
2. Stir in lemon juice, salt, and pepper until well mixed.
3. Serve at room temperature or chill in the refrigerator for at least 1 hour before serving.

Garden Orchard Salad

Fresh veggies, peanuts, and apples give this crunchy salad a refreshing flavor, and it is coated with non-fat vanilla yogurt for creaminess.

Calories: 106 per serving

Makes 4 servings

Ingredients

- 1 1/2 cups broccoli florets (coarsely chopped)
- 1/2 cup carrots (grated)
- 1/2 cup cauliflower (coarsely chopped)
- 1/2 cup apple (chopped, cored and diced, not peeled)
- 1/4 cup green onion (sliced)
- 1/2 cup yogurt, non-fat vanilla
- 1/4 cup peanuts, unsalted, dry-roasted (chopped)

Directions

1. Wash your hands and work area.
2. Mix all ingredients together in serving bowl.
3. Cover and refrigerate for 2 hours or longer to allow flavors to blend. Serve cold.
4. Cover and refrigerate leftovers within 2 hours.

3-Can Chili

With almost no cooking required to prepare this chili, just open cans of beans, corn, and tomatoes, and heat everything together in a pan!

Calories: 129 per serving

Makes 6 servings

Ingredients

- 1 can beans, low-sodium undrained (pinto, kidney, red, or black 15.5 ounces)
- 1 can corn, drained (15 ounces, or 10-ounce package of frozen corn)
- 1 can crushed tomatoes, undrained (15 ounces)
- chili powder (to taste)

Directions

1. Place the contents of all 3 cans into a pan.
2. Add chili powder to taste.
3. Stir to mix
4. Continue to stir over medium heat until heated thoroughly.
5. Refrigerate leftovers.

Baked Potato Soup

The main ingredient is potato. For a heartier dish, add 2 cups diced cooked chicken or turkey ham.

Calories: 267 per serving

Makes 5 servings

Ingredients

- 2 tablespoons light buttery spread

- 1 small onion (chopped)

- 2 medium potatoes (baked, peeled and mashed)

- 3 cups prepared instant nonfat dry milk

- 1 can low-sodium chicken broth (about 14.5 ounces)

- 1 cup reduced-fat cheddar cheese (shredded)

- salt and pepper (to taste)

Directions

1. Melt light buttery spread in a large sauce pot over medium heat and add chopped onion, stirring every once in a while until onions are clear.

2. Stir in potatoes, milk and broth; continue to stir until smooth.

3. Bring to a boil over medium heat, stirring every once in a while.

4. Remove from heat and stir in ½ cup cheese. Add pepper and salt to taste. Sprinkle remaining cheese on top and serve.

Notes

Tip: For a heartier dish, add 2 cups diced cooked chicken or turkey ham.

Beef & Vegetable Soup

When you're looking for a wholesome, delicious meal, look no further than this Beef and Vegetable Soup, featuring canned beef broth, carrots, green beans and stewed tomatoes.

Calories: 226 per serving

Makes 6 servings

Ingredients

- 1 tablespoon vegetable oil

- 1 pound lean ground beef

- 1 medium onion, diced

- 2 cloves garlic, minced

- 1 can low sodium beef broth (14.5-ounce can)

- 1 can sliced carrots, drained (14.5-ounce can)

- 1 can no salt added cut green beans (14.5-ounce can)

- 1 can no salt added stewed tomatoes (14.5-ounce can)

- 1 teaspoon dried basil

- 1 cup cooked egg noodles

Directions

1. In 4-quart saucepan over medium-high heat, in hot oil, cook ground beef until well browned on all sides, stirring frequently.

2. With slotted spoon, remove beef to bowl. In drippings remaining in saucepan over medium heat, cook onion and garlic until tender-crisp.

3. Add beef broth, carrots, green beans, stewed tomatoes, basil and ground beef; over high heat, heat to boiling.

4. Reduce heat to low; cover and simmer 10 to 15 minutes to blend flavors, stirring occasionally.

5. Stir in cooked egg noodles.

Black Bean Soup

Calories: 334 per serving

Makes 5 serving

Ingredients

- 2 tablespoons vegetable oil
- 1 Spanish onion
- 2 carrots (diced)
- 2 celery sticks (diced)
- 4 garlic cloves (peeled and minced)
- 1 teaspoon dried basil
- 1 teaspoon dried oregano
- 2 teaspoons chili powder (or more to taste)
- 3 cans 15.5 ounce low-sodium black beans (drained and rinsed in cold water, or use 6 cups cooked (dried) black beans)
- 8 cups water
- 1 cube low sodium chicken bouillon
- 1 lime (juiced)
- plain low-fat yogurt (optional)

Directions

1. Place a soup or stock pot on the stove over medium heat and when it is hot, add the oil. Add an onion, carrots, celery, garlic, basil, oregano, and chili powder and cook about 10 minutes until the onion is soft.

2. Add the beans, water, and bouillon cube and raise the heat to high and bring to a boil. Turn the heat down to low and cook about 2 1/2 hours until the beans are very tender and the mixture is uniform in color.

3. Just before serving, squeeze the juice of 1/4 lime on each serving and a tablespoon of yogurt.

4. Serve right away, or cover and refrigerate up to 5 days.

Brunswick Stew

Calories: 180 per serving

Makes 8 servings

This hearty stew makes 8 servings or you can double it for a crowd. Skip the trip to the grocery store by using fresh leftover cooked chicken or turkey that has been properly stored and handled in addition to canned veggies from your pantry.

Ingredients

- 1 tablespoon vegetable oil
- 1 onion (medium, chopped)
- 2 cups chicken broth, low-sodium
- 2 cups chicken or turkey (cooked, diced and boned)
- 2 cups tomatoes, canned or cooked (low sodium)
- 2 cups lima beans, canned or cooked
- 2 cups whole kernel corn, canned or cooked

Directions

1. Heat oil in a large pan. Add onion and cook in oil until tender.
2. Add all remaining ingredients. Bring to a simmer for 30 minutes at medium-low.
3. Makes 8 servings of about 1 cup each.

Chicken and Dumpling Soup

Calories: 243 per serving

Makes 8 servings

Ingredients

For the Soup:

- 2 tablespoons vegetable oil
- 2 cups carrot, chopped
- 1 cup onion, chopped
- 1 cup celery, chopped, including some leaves
- 8 cups chicken broth, fat free, reduced sodium
- 2 cups cooked chicken breast, shredded
- 1/2 teaspoon black peppercorns
- 1 teaspoon dried thyme
- 2 bay leaves
- 2 cups fresh spinach leaves, coarsely chopped

For the Dumplings:

- 1 cup whole wheat flour
- 1 cup all-purpose flour
- 3/4 cup skim milk
- 1 egg, large

Directions

1. Heat oil in Dutch oven or soup kettle over medium-high heat.
2. Sauté carrot, onion and celery for 5 minutes; stir in broth, chicken, peppercorns, thyme and bay leaves.
3. Reduce heat to low; simmer, partially covered for 20 minutes.
4. Meanwhile, in small bowl, mix dumpling ingredients until well blended.
5. Drop small spoonfuls of dumpling dough into simmering soup.
6. Cover soup and allow dumplings to cook for about 20 minutes
7. Stir in spinach.
8. Remove bay leaves before serving soup.

Chicken Noodle Soup

Calories: 287 per serving

Makes 6 servings

Ingredients

- 1 pound chicken breasts (thawed, skin and bone removed from each piece)
- 6 cups water
- 1/2 teaspoon salt
- 1/4 teaspoon black pepper
- 4 tablespoons egg mix
- 2 cups all-purpose flour

Directions

1. Cut up chicken breasts and place in a large pot with enough water to cover. Add salt and pepper.

2. Bring chicken and water to a boil. Reduce to medium heat and continue to cook for about 20 minutes.

3. Set aside 1/4 cup (about 1 ladle full) of the broth in a large bowl to cool down.

4. To make the noodles, combine egg mix and flour in a medium-size bowl. While mixing the egg and flour, slowly add the 1/4 cup cooled broth until a dough is formed.

5. Roll the dough on a clean, dry, floured surface. Add more flour as needed to keep it from sticking.

6. Cut dough into 1/2 inch wide strips that are about 6 inches long.

7. Gently put the strips into the pot with the chicken. Stir every 5 minutes.

8. Cook until done (about 15-20 minutes over medium heat). 9. Be careful! Pot may boil over if lid is fully closed.

Cream of Broccoli Soup

This creamy soup makes a perfect lunch or dinner. Keep it healthy using fat-free milk and fresh or frozen broccoli.

Calories: 123 per serving

Makes 4 servings

Ingredients

- 1 1/2 cups chicken broth
- 1/2 cup onion (chopped)
- 2 cups broccoli (cut)
- 1/2 teaspoon thyme (dried, crushed)
- 2 bay leaves (small)
- 2 tablespoons vegetable oil
- 2 tablespoons flour
- 1/4 teaspoon salt
- pepper (dash, optional)
- 1 cup non-fat milk
- garlic powder (dash, optional)

Directions

1. In a saucepan combine chicken broth, chopped onion, broccoli, thyme, bay leaf and garlic powder. Bring mixture to boiling. Reduce heat; cover and simmer for 10 minutes or until vegetables are tender. Remove bay leaf.

2. Place half of the mixture in a blender or food processor, cover and blend 30 to 60 seconds or until smooth. Pour into a bowl; repeat with remaining vegetable mixture, set all aside.

3. In the same saucepan warm the oil. Stir in flour, salt, and pepper. Add the milk all at once, stirring rapidly with a wire whisk. Cook and stir until mixture is thickened and bubbly. Stir in the blended broccoli mixture. Cook and stir until soup is heated through. Season to taste with additional salt and pepper.

Notes

Fresh or frozen broccoli can be used.

Au Gratin Potatoes

One serving of this creamy potato side dish will provide you with half your daily value of vitamin C, almost a quarter of your daily value of fiber, and some calcium and iron.

Calories: 277 per serving

Makes 8 servings

Ingredients

- 6 russet potatoes (medium, 3-4 inch, peeled and sliced into 1/4 inch slices)
- 1 cup onion (chopped)
- 2 tablespoons margarine
- 4 tablespoons flour
- 1 teaspoon salt
- 1 dash black pepper
- 1 1/2 cups cheddar cheese, mild shredded
- 2 cups milk, non-fat

Directions

1. Prepare a large casserole baking pan by coating lightly with oil or cooking oil spray.

2. Make a white sauce by melting margarine in a small pan. Stir in flour. Gradually add milk, stirring constantly.

3. Cook, stirring constantly, until slightly thickened. Remove from heat. Stir in cheese until melted and smooth.

4. Add salt and pepper.

5. Place a layer of potatoes and onion in a prepared casserole pan, using approximately 1/4 of the potatoes and 1/4 cup onion.

6. Spread with 1/2 cup of the sauce prepared in steps 2 and 3.

7. Repeat layers, making a total of 4.

8. Bake at 350 degrees for one hour.

Autumn Vegetable Succotash

This medley of vegetables mixes fresh and frozen vegetables for a side dish that takes a short time to prepare.

Calories: 203 per serving

Makes 8 servings

Ingredients

- 1/4 cup olive oil

- 1 cup onion (diced)

- 2 garlic clove (finely chopped)

- 2 cups bell pepper (red, diced)

- 2 cups zucchini (diced)

- 2 cups summer squash (yellow, diced)

- 3 cups lima beans (frozen)

- 3 cups corn kernels (frozen)

- 2 teaspoons sage, dried (or 2 Tablespoons fresh, coarsely chopped)

Directions

1. In a skillet over medium-high heat, add oil

2. Add onion; cook until translucent (2 minutes). Add garlic, bell peppers, zucchini, squash, lima beans, and corn.

3. Season as desired; cook, stirring, until vegetables are tender (10 minutes). Stir in sage and serve.

Baked Beans

Double or triple this easy recipe to feed a crowd. It's perfect for a picnic or potluck.

Calories: 226 per serving

Makes 6 servings

Ingredients

- 1 1/2 cups navy, kidney or lima beans (dry, sorted and rinsed)
- 2 cups water
- 2 cups apple juice
- 1 teaspoon salt
- 2 tablespoons molasses
- 1/2 cup ketchup
- 2 teaspoons vinegar
- 1 teaspoon mustard (dried)

Directions

1. Combine apple juice and water. Bring to a boil.
2. Add beans and simmer for 2 1/2 hours until beans are tender.
3. Drain beans, reserve the liquid.
4. Put beans and other ingredients in greased baking dish.
5. Cover and bake at 250° for 3 to 4 hours.
6. Uncover the last hour of baking and add some reserved liquid if beans become dry.

Baked Potatoes Primavera

A simple primavera sauce mixed with frozen vegetables takes baked potatoes to a new level.

Calories: 342 per serving

Makes 4 servings

Ingredients

- 4 potatoes (medium)

- 4 cups mixed vegetables (frozen)

- 1 1/4 cups sour cream, non-fat

- 1/2 teaspoon oregano (dried)

- 1/2 teaspoon basil (dried)

- black pepper (to taste)

Directions

1. Pierce each potato several times with a fork. Microwave on high until tender, about 3-4 minutes per potato.

2. Steam mixed vegetables until hot.

3. Mix the sour cream with the herbs and pepper.

4. Split the potatoes in the center and fill with steamed veggies. Top with sour cream and serve hot.

Barley Pilaf

Using quick-cooking barley will cut this recipe time in half. See the notes for more information.

Calories: 119 per serving

Makes 8 servings

Ingredients

- 1 tablespoon vegetable oil

- 1 cup onion (chopped)

- 1/2 cup celery (chopped)

- green or red bell pepper, chopped (1/2 cup, optional)

- 1 cup mushrooms (fresh sliced, or 1- 4 ounce can mushrooms, drained)

- 1 cup pearl barley (uncooked)

- 1 teaspoon vegetable bouillon (or beef or chicken, low sodium)

Directions

1. Place a medium pan over medium heat; add vegetable oil, onion and celery. Cook, stirring often until onion is soft.

2. Add bell pepper (if using), mushrooms and pearl barley. Stir well.

3. Add water and bouillon and stir to dissolve bouillon. Bring to a boil, lower heat and cover pan.

4. Cook for 50 to 60 minutes or until barley is tender and liquid is absorbed.

Black Beans and Rice

This recipe features canned, low-sodium black beans. Serve black beans heated, without adding salt, or use in casseroles, soups, or baked bean dishes.

Calories: 180 per serving

Makes 4 servings

Ingredients

- 1 teaspoon vegetable oil
- 1 tablespoon garlic (finely chopped)
- 1 cup onion (chopped)
- 1 cup green pepper (diced)
- 2 cans low-sodium black beans
- 2 cups low-sodium chicken broth
- 1 tablespoon vinegar
- 1/2 teaspoon oregano
- 3 cups cooked rice
- black pepper to taste

Directions

1. In a large skillet, heat oil and cook garlic, onions, and green peppers for about 3 minutes.

2. Stir in the beans, broth, vinegar, and seasonings and boil.

3. Reduce heat and cover. Cook on low heat for 5 minutes.

4. Spoon over cooked rice and serve.

Broccoli and Corn Bake

This recipe will help you make half your plate fruits and vegetables. Serve this broccoli and corn dish warm at any meal.

Calories: 214 per serving

Makes 6 servings

Ingredients

- 1 can cream-style corn (14.75 ounce)

- 3 3/4 cups broccoli (frozen, cooked)

- 1 egg (beaten)

- 1/2 cup cracker crumbs (crushed)

- 1/4 cup vegetable oil

- 6 saltine crackers (crushed)

- 1 tablespoon tub margarine (or butter) (melted)

Directions

1. Mix corn, broccoli, egg, cracker crumbs and oil together in greased 1 1/2 quart casserole.

2. Mix topping ingredients together in small bowl. Sprinkle over corn mixture.

3. Bake at 350 degrees for 40 minutes.

Brussels Sprouts with Mushroom Sauce

This side dish is delicious when made with brussels sprouts, and you could also make it with broccoli, cabbage, kale, collards, or turnips. Cooking time may vary for different types of vegetables.

Calories: 54 per serving

Makes 2 servings

Ingredients

- 2 cups brussels sprouts (or broccoli, cabbage, kale, collards, or turnips)

- 1/2 cup chicken broth, low-sodium

- 1 teaspoon lemon juice

- 1 teaspoon brown mustard (spicy)

- 1/2 teaspoon thyme (dried)

- 1/2 cup mushroom (sliced)

Directions

1. Trim brussels sprouts and cut in half. Steam until tender - about 6 to 10 minutes, or microwave on high for 3 to 4 minutes.

2. In a non-stick pot bring the broth to a boil.

3. Mix in the lemon juice, mustard, and thyme. Add the mushrooms.

4. Boil until the broth is reduced by half, about 5 to 8 minutes.

5. Add the brussels sprouts (or other cooked vegetable).

6. Toss well to coat with the sauce.

Cauliflower Shells with Cheese

Creamy cauliflower and low-fat cheese make a delicious sauce for this pasta dish.

Calories: 408 per serving

Makes 7 servings

Ingredients

- 1 pound whole wheat pasta shells

- 8 cups water

- 2 cups chopped cauliflower

- 1 1/2 cups milk, non-fat

- 1 teaspoon garlic salt

- 1 cup flour

- 1/4 cup vegetable oil

- 1 cup cheese, low-fat

Directions

1. Fill 1 pot with 6 cups of water and bring to a boil. Once the water is boiling, add pasta and cook for 8 minutes.

2. Drain pasta and fill the same pot with 2 cups of water, bring to a boil.

3. Place the chopped cauliflower in the boiling water and cook until the florets are soft (about 4 minutes). Drain cauliflower.

4. Placed the cooked cauliflower, 1/2 cup milk, and garlic salt in a blender and blend until smooth.

5. In a separate pot, heat oil. Add the flour and whisk until the mixture is smooth. Add 1 cup of milk and cook the mixture until it bubbles and thickens. Add the cheese and cauliflower and mix.

6. Once the mixture is complete, remove from heat. Add the pasta back into the sauce and serve.

15-Minute Enchiladas

This is quick to make. When you need a main dish right away, try this enchilada recipe.

Calories: 410 per serving

Makes 8 servings

Ingredients

- nonstick cooking spray

- 3 cups chili without beans (1 can, about 24 ounces)

- 1 1/2 cups canned refried beans, low-sodium, non-fat

- 2 cups low-fat Cheddar or Monterey jack cheese (shredded)

- 8 flour tortillas, large size

Directions

1. Preheat oven to 350 degrees F.

2. Cover a cookie sheet with foil and spray with nonstick cooking spray.

3. In a medium-size saucepan, heat chili and refried beans until warm (do not boil).

4. Spoon about half of the chili mixture evenly onto the tortillas, sprinkle with cheese, and roll up. Place side by side on the cookie sheet with seam side down.

5. Top tortillas with remaining chili mixture. Sprinkle with remaining cheese.

6. Bake for 10 minutes until cheese is melted.

2-Step Chicken

The ultimate in simplicity, this recipe calls for chicken and cream of chicken soup. Pair it with a salad, rice dish, or steamed vegetables for a complete dinner. Even better, 2-step around the kitchen while it is heating up, getting some physical activity while you cook!

Calories: 181 per serving

Makes 4 servings

Ingredients

- 1 tablespoon vegetable oil

- 2 Boneless chicken breasts

- 1 can cream of chicken soup (10 ounces)

- 1/2 cup water

Directions

1. Heat oil in a skillet at a medium-high setting.

2. Add chicken and cook for ten minutes.

3. Remove chicken from pan and set aside.

4. Stir the soup and water together in the skillet and heat it to a boil.

5. Return the chicken to the skillet. Reduce the heat to low and simmer for an additional 10 minutes, or until the chicken reaches an internal temperature of 165°F.

Notes

To lower sodium content, use reduced sodium cream of chicken soup.

Fancy Fish Tacos

Calories: 393 per serving

Makes 4 servings

Ingredients

- 4 fresh or frozen tilapia fillets

- Salt to taste

- 1 cup quinoa, rinsed

- 1 large carrot, peeled and thinly sliced

- 1 large cucumber, thinly sliced

- 1/2 cup red cabbage

- 1 cup broccoli, chopped

- 1/4 cup fresh cilantro

- 1 juice of 1 lime

- 4 whole-wheat tortillas or wraps

Directions

1. Preheat the oven to 350°F. On a large baking sheet, place the tilapia, and add salt to taste (if frozen, defrost the fish first). Bake for 25 minutes, or until the fish flakes easily with a fork.

2. Meanwhile, in a medium pot, bring 2 cups of water and the quinoa to a boil over medium heat; reduce heat to low and cook for about 20 minutes, or until tender.

3. In a large bowl, combine the vegetables and cilantro. When the fish is done, squeeze lime juice over each fillet. Fill each whole-wheat tortilla with fish and about ¼ cup vegetables. Roll up and serve.

Anytime Pizza

Make your own pizza topped with green peppers, mushrooms, or other vegetables.

Calories: 180 per serving

Makes 2 servings

Ingredients

- 1/4 mini baguette or Italian bread (split lengthwise, or 2 split English muffins)
- 1/2 cup pizza sauce
- 1/2 cup mozzarella or cheddar cheese (part-skim, shredded)
- 1/4 cup green pepper (chopped)
- 1/4 cup mushrooms (fresh or canned, sliced)
- vegetable toppings (other, as desired, optional)
- Italian seasoning (optional)

Directions

1. Toast the bread or English muffin until slightly brown.
2. Top bread or muffin with pizza sauce, vegetables and low-fat cheese.
3. Sprinkle with Italian seasonings as desired.
4. Return bread to toaster oven (or regular oven preheated to 350 degrees).
5. Heat until cheese melts.

Apricot & Lemon Chicken

Why wait for dessert to enjoy your fruit? Make it a part of your meal in this main dish.

Calories: 241 per serving

Makes 4 servings

Ingredients

- 4 chicken breasts, boneless & skinless (medium)

- 1 teaspoon cumin

- 5 tablespoons apricot spread (about 1/3 cup)

- 1 fresh lemon, juiced

- 2 tablespoons water

Directions

1. Rub cumin over chicken and place in skillet.

2. Cook on medium-high for 6 minutes on each side, or until cooked through. Remove from pan and keep warm.

3. Add apricot spread, lemon juice, and water to skillet. On medium heat, stir until smooth.

4. Spoon sauce over chicken and serve warm.

Notes

May substitute approximately 3 Tablespoons of lemon juice for 1 fresh lemon, juiced.

Arroz Con Pollo

This one skillet meal makes a quick, tasty, and healthy weeknight dinner.

Calories: 336 per serving

Makes 4 servings

Ingredients

- 4 6-ounce chicken thighs (bone-in, skin removed)
- 1/2 teaspoon Kosher salt
- 1/2 teaspoon black pepper
- 1 yellow onion (peeled and chopped)
- 1 bell pepper (cored, seeded, and chopped)
- 3 garlic cloves (peeled and minced)
- 1 teaspoon ground cumin
- 1 teaspoon dried oregano
- 1 cup long-grain white rice (uncooked)
- 1 can 14.5 ounce low-sodium diced tomatoes (including liquid)
- 2 cups water
- 1 cube low sodium chicken bouillon

Directions

1. Place the skillet over medium high heat and when it is hot, add the chicken thighs, skin side down and cook until browned, then flip, about 5 minutes on each side.

2. Turn the heat off, carefully remove the chicken from the skillet and transfer to the plate. Pour off all but 1 tablespoon fat.

3. Reheat the skillet over low heat and add the onion, pepper, garlic, cumin, and oregano and cook until the onion is softened, about 10 minutes.

4. Add the uncooked rice and tomatoes and stir well.

5. Add the water and bouillon cube and bring to a boil over high heat. Return chicken to pan, skin side down, turn the heat down to low and cover.

6. Cook chicken for 20 minutes and then carefully flip so that the skin side is up.

7. Cover and cook for an additional 20 minutes. Serve right away.

Baked Chicken with Vegetables

Roast carrots, potatoes, and onion are cooked along with chicken for a complete oven-baked meal.

Calories: 485 per serving

Makes 4 servings

Ingredients

- 4 potatoes (sliced)

- 6 carrot (sliced)

- 1 onion (large, quartered)

- 1 chicken (raw, - cut into pieces, skin removed)

- 1/2 cup water

- 1 teaspoon thyme

- 1/4 teaspoon pepper

Directions

1. Preheat oven to 400 degrees.

2. Place potatoes, carrots and onions in a large roasting pan.

3. Put chicken pieces on top of the vegetables.

4. Mix water, thyme and pepper. Pour over chicken and vegetables.

5. Spoon juices over chicken once or twice during cooking.

6. Bake at 400 degrees for one hour or more until browned and tender.

Baked Fish and Vegetables

Frozen fish is a good option when you need a quick meal. Wrap it up in some foil with vegetables and bake for only 10 minutes!

Calories: 145 per serving

Makes 4 servings

Ingredients

- 4 4-ounce white fish fillets (frozen, or cod or perch)
- 2 cups mixed vegetables (frozen)
- 1 onion (small, diced)
- 1 teaspoon lemon juice (or fresh lemon, sliced thin)
- 1 tablespoon parsley flakes (dried or fresh chopped)
- aluminum foil

Directions

1. Preheat oven to 450 degrees.
2. Separate and place fish fillets in center of each tin foil square.
3. Combine frozen vegetables and diced onion in bowl and mix. Spoon vegetables around fillets.
4. Sprinkle with lemon juice (or top with lemon slice) and add parsley on top. Fold ends of tin foil together to form leak-proof seal.
5. Bake for 10 minutes. Serve.

Baked Lemon Chicken

Lemon, onions, and thyme decorate this oven-baked chicken.

Calories: 261 per serving

Makes 5 servings

Ingredients

- 3 1/2 pounds chicken (skinned and cut into 10 pieces)
- 1/4 teaspoon salt
- 1/4 teaspoon pepper
- 1 1/2 cloves of garlic (thinly sliced, or 1 tsp garlic powder)
- 4 teaspoons thyme sprigs (4 fresh sprigs, or 1 tsp dried thyme)
- 3 cups onion (thinly sliced)
- 1 1/2 cups chicken stock (or water)
- 1/4 cup lemon juice
- 1 lemon (sliced into 10 slices, seeds removed)

Directions

1. Combine salt, pepper, garlic, and thyme.
2. Lay chicken pieces into a 11x13 baking pan. Sprinkle seasonings over chicken.
3. Combine onions, stock, and lemon juice in a sauce pan. Heat to a boil.
4. Pour hot lemon mixtue around chicken. Top each chicken piece with a lemon slice.
5. Bake for 30 minutes at 400 degrees until golden brown and juices are clear colored.

Baked Meatballs

Make your own meatballs to use now or freeze them for a quick dinner at another time.

Calories: 131 per serving

Makes: 8 servings (3 meatballs)

Ingredients

- 1 pound ground beef, 90% lean (or ground turkey)
- 1 egg
- 1/2 teaspoon dried parsley
- 1/2 cup bread crumbs
- 1/2 cup milk, 1% (or non-fat)
- 1/4 teaspoon pepper
- 1 teaspoon onion powder

Directions

1. Mix all ingredients, shape into balls (about 24 meatballs)
2. Arrange on baking sheets that have been sprayed with non-stick cooking spray.
3. Bake at 425°F for 12-15 minutes. It is best to use a food safety thermometer to check for doneness (it should read 160°F for ground beef and 165°F for ground turkey).
4. If meatballs are being saved for future use, chill rapidly; package in amounts needed per meal and freeze immediately.

Baked Pork Chops

Green and red peppers top these festive pork chops.

Calories: 225 per serving

Makes: 6 servings

Ingredients

- 6 pork chops (lean center-cut, 1/2-inch thick)
- 1 onion (medium, thinly sliced)
- 1/2 cup green pepper (chopped)
- 1/2 cup red pepper (chopped)
- 1/8 teaspoon black pepper
- 1/4 teaspoon salt

Directions

1. Preheat oven to 375 degrees.

2. Trim fat from pork chops. Place chops in a 13x9-inch baking pan.

3. Spread onion and peppers on top of chops. Sprinkle with pepper and salt. Refrigerate for 1 hour.

4. Cover pan and cook 30 minutes.

5. Uncover, turn chops and re-cover with onions and peppers, and continue cooking for an additional 15 minutes or until internal temperature reaches 145 degrees. Garnish with fresh parsley.

Barbecue Beef

This recipe is delicious on its own, served with either rice or potatoes and vegetables. Or try spooning the cooked beef onto a sandwich roll.

Calories: 390 per serving

Makes: 8 Servings

Ingredients

- 1 frozen beef roast (2 pounds, thawed)

- 4 cloves garlic (chopped)

- 1/2 teaspoon black pepper

- 1 1/2 cups barbecue sauce

Directions

1. Preheat oven to 425 degrees F.

2. Place beef roast in a roasting pan. Rub garlic and pepper on the roast and put in the oven for 30 minutes.

3. Turn oven down to 325 degrees F, and roast another 2 to 3 hours or until beef is tender enough to be pulled apart with a fork.

4. Remove from oven. Shred beef by pulling it apart with a fork into a bowl.

5. Pour barbecue sauce and garlic over beef. Stir well.

Bean and Rice Burritos

These baked burritos are a great way to use leftover cooked rice. Try them with brown rice for a whole grain boost.

Calories: 358 per serving

Makes: 8 servings

Ingredients

- 2 cups rice (cooked)

- 1 onion (small, chopped)

- 2 cups kidney beans (cooked, or one 15 ounce can, drained)

- 8 flour tortillas (10 inch)

- 1/2 cup salsa

- 1/2 cup cheese (shredded)

Directions

1. Preheat the oven to 300 degrees.

2. Peel the onion, and chop it into small pieces.

3. Drain the liquid from the cooked (or canned) kidney beans.

4. Mix the rice, chopped onion, and beans in a bowl.

5. Put each tortilla on a flat surface.

6. Put 1/2 cup of the rice and bean mix in the middle of each tortilla.

7. Fold the sides of the tortilla to hold the rice and beans.

8. Put each filled tortilla (burrito) in the baking pan.

9. Bake for 15 minutes.

10. While the burritos are baking, grate 1/2 cup cheese.

11. Pour the salsa over the baked burritos. Add cheese.

Beef & Noodles

This protein-filled dinner makes it easy to put food on the table even when you're short on ingredients. Serve it with cooked vegetables from the freezer for a complete meal.

Calories: 224 per serving

Makes 4 Servings

Ingredients

- 3/4 pound ground beef, 85% lean

- 1 1/2 cups water (can take up to 2 cups water)

- 2 cups egg noodles, uncooked (or any shaped pasta)

- 7 Servings Eating Smart Seasoning Mix

- salt (optional)

Directions

1. Brown 3/4 pound ground beef in a large skillet, drain the fat.

2. Add water, egg noodles or pasta, and seasoning mix. Stir.

3. Bring to a boil, reduce heat to low and simmer covered for 15-20 minutes or until noodles are tender.

4. Taste; then add a small amount of salt, if needed.

5. Refrigerate leftovers.

Black Bean Burgers

Black beans and cooked rice are used as the base of these delicious burgers. Flavored with scallions, garlic and spices, these are sure to please the whole family.

Calories: 274 per serving

Makes 4 Servings

Ingredients

- 1 can 15.5 ounce low-sodium black beans (drained and rinsed).
- 1 large egg
- 1/2 cup cooked brown rice
- 2 scallions (green and white minced about 1/4 cup)
- 2 tablespoons Chopped fresh cilantro (or basil leaves or a combination)
- 1 clove garlic (peeled and minced)
- 1/4 teaspoon dried oregano or basil
- 1 teaspoon vegetable oil
- 1/2 teaspoon salt
- 1/2 teaspoon black pepper
- 4 whole-wheat buns

Directions

1. Add beans to a bowl and mash with a fork until chunky. Add the egg and mix well.

2. Add precooked rice, scallions, garlic and oregano, salt and pepper and mix until well combined.

3. Divide the mixture into 4 portions and form each portion into a patty about ¾ to 1 inch thick.

4. Place a large skillet on the stove on high heat. When the skillet is hot, add oil. Add burgers and cook 4 to 5 minutes per side until browned on both sides and heated throughout. Place on a whole wheat bun.

Broccoli Alfredo

This dish features whole wheat pasta and fat-free Parmesan cheese.

Calories: 324 per serving

Makes: 4 Servings

Ingredients

- 4 cups broccoli, cooked
- 4 cups cooked whole wheat pasta
- 2 cups milk, 1% (or non-fat)
- 1 cup parmesan cheese (reduced fat)
- 1 teaspoon basil
- 1/2 teaspoon garlic powder
- 2 tablespoons cornstarch
- pepper (to taste, optional)

Directions

1. Heat milk over medium heat and then add basil and garlic powder. When hot, add Parmesan cheese.

2. Mix cornstarch with 2 or 3 Tbsp of milk and add to hot mixture. Heat until thickened.

3. Pour mixture over pasta and broccoli. Serve.

Cheesy Chicken, Broccoli and Rice Bake

A great recipe to use leftover chicken that has been properly handled combined with broccoli, cheese, onions, garlic, and brown rice to create a quick dinner.

Calories: 239 per serving

Makes: 12 servings

Ingredients

- 5 cups water
- 2 1/2 cups rice
- 1/4 cup onion (chopped)
- 1 garlic clove (chopped)
- 1 cup milk (skim)
- 1 can cream of mushroom soup (10.75 ounces, condensed, 98% fat-free)
- 1/4 teaspoon salt
- 1/4 teaspoon pepper
- 3/4 cup cheddar cheese, low-fat (grated)
- 2 cups chicken (shredded, cooked)
- 2 cups broccoli (pieces)

Directions

1. Preheat oven to 350° F. In large saucepan bring water to boil. Add rice, onion, and garlic. Cook for about 20 minutes or until rice is soft.

2. While rice is cooking combine milk, soup, salt, and pepper, mix well. When rice is done combine with milk mixture, chicken and broccoli, mix well.

3. Grease 9 x 13 pan and pour mixture into pan. Bake in the preheated oven for 18 minutes. Sprinkle with cheese. Bake for another 6 minutes or until cheese is melted. Serve immediately.

Chicken Spaghetti

This colorful crowd-pleaser that incorporates vegetables, whole grains, protein and dairy in one dish. Serve with some fresh, frozen, canned, or dried fruit for a meal that contains all of the food groups.

Calories: 363 per serving

Makes 4 servings

Ingredients

- vegetable oil spray
- 4 ounces spaghetti, whole wheat uncooked
- 1 teaspoon olive oil
- 1 red bell pepper, medium (thinly sliced)
- 1 green bell pepper, medium (thinly sliced)
- 1 onion, medium (chopped)
- 2 cups cooked chicken breast, skinless and diced (cooked without salt, about 8 ounces)
- 1 can tomatoes, diced undrained (14.5 ounces) (low sodium)
- 1 can cream of chicken soup (reduced sodium (10.75 ounces))
- 1/2 cup cheddar cheese, reduced fat shredded
- 1/4 cup Parmesan cheese (shredded or grated)
- 1/4 teaspoon pepper

Directions

1. Preheat the oven to 350°F. Lightly spray an 8-inch square baking dish with vegetable oil spray.

2. Prepare the spaghetti using the package directions, omitting the salt and oil. Drain well in a colander.

3. Meanwhile, in a large skillet, heat the oil over medium heat, swirling to coat the bottom. Cook the bell peppers and onion for 4 to 5 minutes, or until tender, stirring occasionally.

4. Pour into a large bowl. Stir in the remaining ingredients, including the spaghetti. Pour into a baking dish.

5. Bake, covered, for 20 minutes. Bake, uncovered for 10 minutes, or until the mixture is warmed through and light golden brown on top.

Chili Tomato Macaroni

You don't have to use salt in this macaroni, tomato, and beef dish seasoned with the Eating Smart Seasoning Mix.

Calories: 329 per serving

Makes 4 Servings

Ingredients

- 3/4 pound ground beef, 85% lean

- 1 1/2 cups water

- 1 cup macaroni, uncooked

- 1 can diced tomatoes, drained (15 ounces)

- 2 teaspoons chili powder, mild

- 8 Servings Eating Smart Seasoning Mix

- salt (optional, to taste)

Directions

1. Brown ground beef in a large skillet, drain the fat.

2. Add water, macaroni, tomatoes, chili powder, and seasoning mix. Stir.

3. Bring to a boil, reduce heat to low and simmer covered on low heat for 20 minutes or until macaroni is tender.

4. Taste; add a small amount of salt if needed.

5. Refrigerate leftovers.

Colorful Quesadillas

Use fresh or frozen spinach and red peppers, or try adding your own colorful vegetables in this dish.

Calories: 156 per serving

Makes: 8 servings

Ingredients

- 8 ounces cream cheese, fat-free

- 1/4 teaspoon garlic powder

- 8 flour tortillas (6" across)

- 1 cup sweet red pepper (chopped)

- 1 cup low-fat cheese (shredded)

- 2 cups spinach leaves (fresh, or 9 oz. frozen, thawed and squeezed dry)

Directions

1. In a small bowl, mix the cream cheese and garlic powder.

2. Spread about 2 tablespoons of the cheese mixture on each tortilla.

3. Sprinkle about 2 tablespoons bell pepper and 2 tablespoons cheese on one half of each tortilla.

4. Add spinach: 1/4 cup if using fresh leaves OR 2 Tablespoons if using frozen. Fold tortillas in half.

5. Heat a large skillet over medium heat until hot. Put 2 folded tortillas in skillet and heat for 1-2 minutes on each side or until golden brown.

6. Remove quesadillas from skillet, place on platter and cover with foil to keep warm while cooking the remainder.

7. Cut each quesadilla into 4 wedges. Serve warm.

Red Beans and Rice

This flavorful dish is traditionally eaten on Monday nights in many homes and uses dry beans, onion, pepper, and spices.

Calories: 232 per serving

Makes 8 servings

Ingredients

- cooking oil spray, as needed (non-stick)
- 1 onion (medium, peeled and chopped)
- 1 green bell pepper (medium, washed, seeded and chopped)
- 1 teaspoon garlic powder
- 2 cans diced tomatoes (14.5 ounces each)
- 1 can kidney beans (15.5 oz, drained and rinsed)
- 6 cups cooked brown rice

Directions

1. Spray skillet with cooking oil spray.
2. Cook onion and pepper over medium heat for 5 minutes or until tender.
3. Add garlic powder, tomatoes, and kidney beans.
4. Bring mixture to a boil.
5. Reduce heat to low and simmer for 5 minutes.
6. Serve over rice.

Jamaican Jerk Chicken

Turn up the heat with this spicy and savory chicken dish! Packed with aromatics and spices this chicken dish is bursting with flavor! Serve with a side of rice and a fresh tossed salad.

Calories: 150 per serving

Makes 10 servings

Ingredients

- 1/2 teaspoon cinnamon (ground)
- 1 1/2 teaspoons allspice (ground)
- 1 1/2 teaspoons black pepper (ground)
- 1 teaspoon hot pepper (crushed, dried)
- 2 teaspoons oregano (crushed)
- 1 teaspoon hot pepper (chopped)
- 1 teaspoon thyme
- 1/2 teaspoon salt
- 6 garlic clove (finely chopped)
- 1 cup onion (pureed or finely chopped)
- 1/4 cup vinegar
- 3 teaspoons brown sugar
- 8 pieces of chicken, skinless (4 drumsticks, 4 breasts)

Directions

1. Preheat oven to 350 degrees Fahrenheit.

2. Combine all ingredients except chicken in large bowl. Rub seasonings over chicken and marinate in refrigerator for 6 hours or longer.

3. Space chicken evenly on non-stick or lightly greased baking pan.

4. Cover with aluminum foil and bake for 40 minutes. Remove foil and continue baking for an additional 30–40 minutes or until the meat can easily be pulled away from the bone with a fork.

Easy Meatloaf

This meatloaf is very moist and simple to make for lunch or dinner. Serve with vegetables, rice, pasta, or potatoes, or slice to make sandwiches.

Calories: 292 per serving

Makes 6 Servings

Ingredients

- 1 pound ground beef
- 1 can low-sodium cream style corn (about 15 ounces)
- 1/2 cup onion (diced)
- 1 teaspoon garlic (finely chopped)
- 1/2 cup water
- 1/2 cup cornmeal
- 2 tablespoons egg mix
- 1/4 teaspoon salt
- 1/4 teaspoon black pepper
- nonstick cooking spray

Directions

1. Preheat oven to 375 degrees F.

2. In a large pan, cook ground beef over medium heat for 8 to 10 minutes. Drain fat.

3. Add corn, onions, and garlic to pan, and cook for an additional 10 minutes.

4. Add water, cornmeal, egg mix, salt, and pepper to the beef mixture. Stir well and cook for 15 minutes.

5. Use a large iron skillet or loaf pan. Spray pan with nonstick cooking spray. Form beef and cornmeal mixture into a loaf in a pan.

6. Cover pan with an oven-safe lid or foil and bake for 35 to 40 minutes.

Mushroom Beef Sloppy Joe's

Chopped mushrooms, when sautéed, blend seamlessly with ground meats. Swapping or adding mushrooms to a recipe can add an extra serving of vegetables to the plate.

Calories: 230 per serving

Makes: 4 Servings

Ingredients

- 1/2 pound white button mushrooms
- 1/2 pound cremini mushrooms
- 1/4 pound 90% lean ground beef
- 1 1/2 tablespoons canola oil
- 1/2 cup chopped onion
- 1 clove garlic (minced)
- 1 can 8oz no-salt-added tomato sauce
- 1 tablespoon chili powder
- 3 teaspoons brown sugar
- 1 teaspoon cider vinegar
- 1/8 teaspoon ground black pepper
- 4 whole-wheat buns

Directions

1. Chop mushrooms to approximate size and texture of ground beef.

2. Heat a sauté pan over medium-high heat.

3. Add ground beef and mushrooms, and cook.

4. Sauté until ground beef is done.

5. Remove mushroom-beef mixture from pan.

6. Add onions and garlic to pan; cook until golden.

7. Return mushroom-beef mixture to pan, along with remaining ingredients.

8. Simmer about 10 minutes; remove from heat.

Orange and Honey Glazed Pork Chops

Broil your chops, instead of pan-frying to reduce fat and calorie. Add zest with the orange juice called for in this recipe.

Calories: 265 per serving

Makes 4 Servings

Ingredients

- 4 Boneless Pork Chops

- 1/4 cup honey

- 1/3 cup orange juice

- 1 tablespoon parsley flakes

- 1 tablespoon garlic pepper seasoning

Directions

1. Sprinkle all sides of chops with garlic pepper seasoning.

2. Broil, 5 to 6 inches from heat, for 6 to 7 minutes per side until internal temperature reaches 150 degrees Fahrenheit.

3. Combine orange juice and honey; brush on pork chop surface; broil 1 minute. Turn and repeat with other side. Sprinkle with parsley before serving.

Pasta Bolognese

This rich red sauce combines ground beef, carrots, celery, onion, tomatoes with a touch of milk for added creaminess.

Calories: 297 per serving

Makes 4 Servings

Ingredients

- 1 tablespoon vegetable oil
- 1 carrot (scrubbed and diced into 1/4-inch pieces)
- 1 celery stalk (chopped into 1/4-inch pieces)
- 1 yellow onion (peeled and chopped into 1/4 inch pieces)
- 3/4 pound lean ground beef (80-85% lean)
- 1 cup water
- 2 cans 14.5-ounce low-sodium crushed or diced tomatoes
- 1/4 cup low-sodium tomato paste
- 1 cup 2% milk
- 8 ounces whole wheat pasta
- 1/4 cup grated Parmesan cheese

Directions

1. Put skillet on the stove over medium heat and when it is hot, add oil. Add carrot, celery, and onion and cook about 10 minutes, stirring occasionally, until the vegetables begin to brown. Raise the heat to high. Pinch off tablespoon-size pieces of the beef and add a few at a time, stirring well between additions. Cook, breaking the meat apart until it is no longer raw, starts to give off liquid, and no longer clumps together, about 10 minutes.

2. Add the water, tomatoes, and tomato paste, stirring well. Cook about 10 minutes until the sauce begins to thicken.

3. Slowly stir in the milk, a little bit at a time. Turn the heat down to low and cook 45 minutes until all the liquid has been absorbed.

4. To cook the pasta: fill a large pot halfway with water. Bring it to a boil over high heat. Add the pasta and about 12 minutes cook until just tender. Drain the pasta and divide into 4 bowls. Top each bowl with about ¾ cup Bolognese and sprinkle with 1 tablespoon Parmesan cheese. Serve right away.

Pineapple Pork

Savory and sweet, delicious pineapple pork chops are a fast and flavorful meal. Enjoy over brown rice or quinoa.

Calories: 285 per serving

Makes 4 servings

Ingredients

- 1 green pepper (medium)
- 4 pork chops (boneless, about 1 pound)
- 1/8 teaspoon salt
- 1 tablespoon vegetable oil
- 1 cup pineapple chunks (8-ounce, undrained)
- 1/4 teaspoon ginger
- 1/4 teaspoon cinnamon

Directions

1. Cut the green pepper into strips.
2. Heat the oil in a large skillet.
3. Place pork chops on the heated skillet. Sprinkle the salt on top.
4. Cook the pork for 5 minutes on low heat on each side.
5. The pork should lose its pink color when it's cooked enough.
6. Remove the cooked pork from the skillet. Place it in a serving dish.
7. Put the green pepper slices in the skillet.
8. Stir the in pineapple chunks with their juice.
9. Stir in the ginger and cinnamon.
10. Simmer for about 3-5 minutes.
11. Spoon the pineapple mixture over cooked pork.

112

Quick Start guide

The Main key to losing weight and maintaining a healthy weight is to consume less calories and become more active. If you are able to accomplish this you will not only find that you will lose weight, but also feel healthier.

This quick start guide is intended to help you get started with your weight-loss goals right away. Each of these steps are important and are crucial to ensuring maximum success, so do your best not to skip any of them.

Below are the 8 steps you will need to take to change your diet and lose weight:

1. **Make a list of goals** – pick three of four things you would like accomplish in the short-term and long-term.

2. **Calculate your BMR** – it will be important to understand how many calories you will be able to take in to lose weight.

3. **Evaluate your physical activities** – Make a list of current activities evaluate how many calories you might burn.

4. **Find food substitutes** – Go through your pantry and refrigerator a try to identify item you know you can find healthier alternatives.

5. **Create a meal plan** – before shopping for food create list of meals for the week and make sure they follow the guidelines of your new diet.

6. **Get rid of your unhealthy foods** – again go through your pantry and refrigerator and look at the foods that you know are not healthy. If you cannot find a healthy alternative throw it out!

7. **Find Encouragement** – find a friend that either has the same goal as you or you know will encourage you to reach your goals. This will be a friend that you know will hold you accountable.

8. **Pick a start date** – choose a day to start and stick with that date. Starting sooner is always better.

1. Make a list of goals

Write down a goal for the week month and an overall goal. They don't have to be weight related goals, they can be size goals, activity related, or even overall health goals. Be sure to reward yourself for reaching a goal! Here are some goals to help you get started:

1.   Weakly Goal – Walk 1 mile

2.   Monthly Goal – Lose 5 lbs.

3.   Overall Goal – Fit into that old dress or pair of pants

These are just some of the goals you could use and we all have our different reasons for wanting to lose weight and become healthier, so decide what has motivated you and try o reach those goals.

After you have made your list of goals decide how you plan to reward yourself, because a goal is not worth working towards unless there is some sort of reward at the end. Make sure the reward has nothing to do with food, but instead maybe something you have always wanted to do.

A reward could be anything big or small and it doesn't have to be anything expensive, just make sure that it is something that you really want and you know will motivate to reach your goals. Some great examples of non-food related rewards include:

- Concert tickets

- A weekend trip or vacation

- Shopping for new clothes

- Manicure and or pedicure

- A round of golf

The possibilities are endless when it comes to goals and rewards, just make sure it is something that will make you happy and motivate you to reach your goals.

2. Calculate your BMR

First to calculate your BMR using the formulas below. This will tell you how many calories you need to consume to maintain your current weight with little to no activity or exercise.

- Women: BMR = 655 + (4.35 x weight in pounds) + (4.7 x height in inches) - (4.7 x age in years)

- Men: BMR = 66 + (6.23 x weight in pounds) + (12.7 x height in inches) - (6.8 x age in years)

Next use the formulas below based on different levels of activity. This will also give you an idea how different levels of activities change the amount of calories you can consume. Multiply your BMR by the appropriate activity factor, as follows:

- Sedentary (little or no exercise): BMR x 1.2

- Lightly active (light exercise/sports 1-3 days/week): BMR x 1.375

- Moderately active (moderate exercise/sports 3-5 days/week): BMR x 1.55

- Very active (hard exercise/sports 6-7 days a week): BMR x 1.725

- Extra active (very hard exercise/sports & physical job or 2x training): BMR x 1.9

Finally multiply your adjusted BMR by .80 to give you the target amount of calories you can consume in order to lose weight. We do not recommend multiplying your adjusted BMR by anything less than .75 or 75% and do not multiply the adjusted BMR by anything greater than 1.00 or 100% unless for some reason you are wanting to gain weight.

3. Pick 3 to 4 physical activities

Make a list of 3 to 4 activities that you enjoy or that are easy to accomplish. Try doing at least one of those activities once every other day. This will give to time to relax in between. On days you don't exercise try replacing some of your activities with physically demanding tasks, like mowing the grass with a push mower or walking to the store in place of driving.

Date	SUN	MON	TUE	WED	THU	FRI	SAT
Exercise	Yoga		Yoga		Walk		Abs
When	In Morning		Before Work		After Dinner		After Work

Start with Walking

We've got the tools and resources to get you on the right path to a healthier lifestyle.

It's Easy

- Walking is the simplest way to start and continue a fitness journey.

- Walking costs nothing to get started.

- Walking is easy and safe.

It Works

- Walking for as few as 30 minutes a day provides heart health benefits.

- Walking is one of the most effective form of exercise to achieve heart health.

And walking isn't your only option. Try these tips for increasing physical activity wherever you are. You may be surprised at all your opportunities to increase your physical activity every day.

4. Find substitutes for high-calorie foods

Look for foods and in your pantry or refrigerator that you know are unhealthy and try to either eliminate them from your diet or replace them with healthier options. It might be easier to pick only three to four foods to start. It will be tough at first to give up some foods especially if it is a food you enjoy, so it might be a good idea to start with foods you don't mind giving up.

After you have chosen the foods you know you need to substitute do some research online to find alternatives. As long as the alternative has less fat and less calories you should be in the clear.

Some examples of foods you should try to substitute:

- Salad dressing – look for low calorie alternatives or possibly make your own

- Pork Bacon – a good alternative to the bacon we all love is turkey bacon. It is both lower in calories and fat.

- Soft Drinks – Its good to eliminate all soft drinks if you can, but if you do decide to have one try a healthier alternative like a sparkling water or diet drink.

- Cheese – while all cheeses are different and in moderation is not bad for you diet, it is one of those foods that you need to find better alternatives to. Try to stay away from processed cheese if possible.

5. Create a meal plan

Start by only consuming *80% of the necessary calories* and dividing those into 3 meals. If you start with smaller meals in the day you can always adjust your remaining meals for an increase in calories consumed. So if you eat a heavy breakfast you can always cut down at lunch and or dinner.

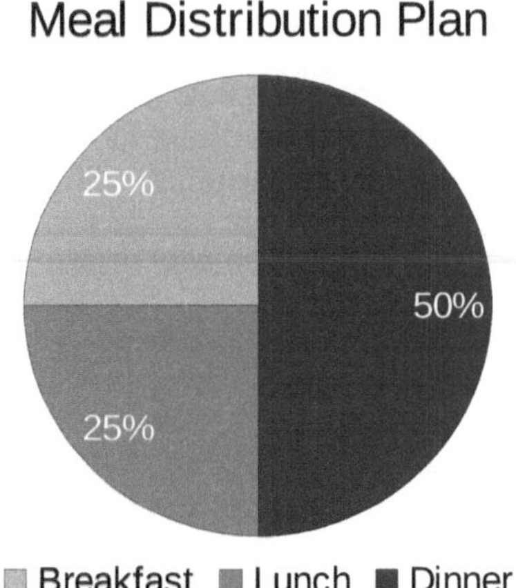

Each meal is a building block in your healthy eating style. Make sure to include all the food groups throughout the day. Make fruits, vegetables, grains, dairy, and protein foods part of your daily meals and snacks. Also, limit added sugars, saturated fat, and sodium. Use a Daily Checklist and the tips below to meet your needs throughout the day.

1. Make half your plate veggies and fruits

Vegetables and fruits are full of nutrients that support good health. Choose fruits and red, orange, and dark-green vegetables such as tomatoes, sweet potatoes, and broccoli.

2. Include whole grains

Aim to make at least half your grains whole grains. Look for the words "100% whole grain" or "100% whole wheat" on the food label. Whole grains provide more nutrients, like fiber, than refined grains.

3. Don't forget the dairy

Complete your meal with a cup of fat-free or low-fat milk. You will get the same amount of calcium and other essential nutrients as whole milk but fewer calories.

4. Add lean protein

Choose protein foods such as lean beef, pork, chicken, or turkey, and eggs, nuts, beans, or tofu. Twice a week, make seafood the protein on your plate.

5. Avoid extra fat

Using heavy gravies or sauces will add fat and calories to otherwise healthy choices. Try steamed broccoli with a sprinkling of low-fat parmesan cheese or a squeeze of lemon.

6. Get creative in the kitchen

Whether you are making a sandwich, a stir-fry, or a casserole, find ways to make them healthier. Try using less meat and cheese, which can be higher in saturated fat and sodium, and adding in more veggies that add new flavors and textures to your meals.

7. Take control of your food

Eat at home more often so you know exactly what you are eating. If you eat out, check and compare the nutrition information. Choose options that are lower in calories, saturated fat, and sodium.

8. Try new foods

Keep it interesting by picking out new foods you've never tried before, like mango, lentils, quinoa, kale, or sardines. You may find a new favorite! Trade fun and tasty recipes with friends or find them online.

9. Satisfy your sweet tooth in a healthy way

Indulge in a naturally sweet dessert dish—fruit! Serve a fresh fruit salad or a fruit parfait made with yogurt. For a hot dessert, bake apples and top with cinnamon.

10. Everything you eat and drink matters

The right mix of foods in your meals and snacks can help you be healthier now and into the future.

6.　Get rid of your junk food

Many of us eat junk food every day. This might be sugar-sweetened drinks like fizzy drinks and high-kilojoule foods like potato chips, dough nuts or French fries. However, your body can't run properly on poor fuel.

Compared to home-cooked food, junk food (which includes fast food) is almost always:

- higher in fat, particularly saturated fat

- higher in salt

- higher in sugar

- lower in fiber

- lower in nutrients, such as calcium and iron

- served in larger portions, which means more calories

Eating too much junk food can leave you feeling sluggish. Eating healthier will boost your vitality and help to keep your skin clear.

Empty Your Refrigerators and Cupboards

Start by making a list of all of the junk food you have in the home and then make another list of healthy alternatives. This will help eliminate the craving of junk food and replaces it with food that is good for you.

After you have made your lists of alternative foods, start throwing away the junk food. This might seem like a waste, but it is not doing anyone any good by staying around. In fact if you don't throw away your junk food you might be tempted to eat it and thats not good either.

Next go shopping for those health alternatives and refrain from purchasing anymore junk food! If you stock your home with only foods that are good for you, you have no other choice but to eat healthy.

7.   Have a Start Date

Old habits die hard. Changing your habits is a process that involves several stages. Sometimes it takes a while before changes become new habits. And, you may face roadblocks along the way.

It might seem like there is never a good time to start your new diet, and this is probably true for most of us. The best thing to do is to start your new plan as soon as possible. Start it today if you can!

Pick a day – You can probably read hundreds of articles around the web from experts that will give you there opinion on which days are best. My opinion is that is important to start as soon as possible no matter and that there is no special day that leads to a more successful transition.

Set Early Goals – Reward yourself early because the first few days and even weeks are important to creating new habits. You want to feel like your making positive even if they are small ones.

Create Accountability – Share your new healthy choices with friends and family members in the hopes that they ask you about your progress. Even if you don't have any progress to share it give them the opportunity to share encouragement.

Do Restart a Diet – If you find yourself slipping from your new diet don't pick a new start date, just continue to make changes to your current habits and identify what caused your lapse in eat-healthy.

If you don't choose to start your date today pick a day to start your new diet in the near future. The longer you wait to start changing your current eating habits the hard it will be to change them in the future. When you do finally pick a day to start stick to it.

122

Helpful Links and Sources

USDA Nutrition.gov - www.nutrition.gov

USDA Food Composition - ndb.nal.usda.gov

U.S. Department of Health & Human Services - www.foodsafety.gov

USDA Choose My Plate - www.choosemyplate.gov

National Agricultural Library Digital Collections - naldc.nal.usda.go

SnapEd Connection - snaped.fns.usda.gov

MedLine Plus - medlineplus.gov/weightcontrol.html

Department of Health & Human Services - www.hhs.gov/fitness/eat-healthy/

ODPHP HealthyPeople.gov - www.healthypeople.gov

ODPHP Health Finder - healthfinder.gov/FindServices

U.S. Food and Drug Administration - www.fda.gov

Australian Dept. of Health - www.eatforhealth.gov.au

American Diabetes Association - http://spectrum.diabetesjournals.org

Australian Dept. of Health - www.healthdirect.gov.au

Australian Dept. of Health - http://www.health.gov.au